T0286890

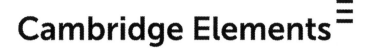

Cambridge Elements

Elements in Child Development
edited by
Marc H. Bornstein
National Institute of Child Health and Human Development, Bethesda
Institute for Fiscal Studies, London
UNICEF, New York City

CHILD DEVELOPMENT IN EVOLUTIONARY PERSPECTIVE

David F. Bjorklund
Florida Atlantic University

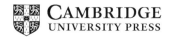

CAMBRIDGE
UNIVERSITY PRESS

University Printing House, Cambridge CB2 8BS, United Kingdom

One Liberty Plaza, 20th Floor, New York, NY 10006, USA

477 Williamstown Road, Port Melbourne, VIC 3207, Australia

314–321, 3rd Floor, Plot 3, Splendor Forum, Jasola District Centre, New Delhi – 110025, India

79 Anson Road, #06–04/06, Singapore 079906

Cambridge University Press is part of the University of Cambridge.

It furthers the University's mission by disseminating knowledge in the pursuit of education, learning, and research at the highest international levels of excellence.

www.cambridge.org
Information on this title: www.cambridge.org/9781108791502
DOI: 10.1017/9781108866187

© David F. Bjorklund 2020

First published 2020

A catalogue record for this publication is available from the British Library.

ISBN 978-1-108-79150-2 Paperback
ISSN 2632–9948 (online)
ISSN 2632-993X (print)

Child Development in Evolutionary Perspective

Elements in Child Development

DOI: 10.1017/9781108866187
First published online: October 2020

David F. Bjorklund
Florida Atlantic University

Author for correspondence: dfbjorklund@gmail.com; dbjorklu@fau.edu

Abstract: Natural selection has operated as strongly or more so on the early stages of the lifespan as on adulthood. One evolved feature of human childhood is high levels of behavioral, cognitive, and neural plasticity, permitting children to adapt to a wide range of physical and social environments. Taking an evolutionary perspective on infancy and childhood provides a better understanding of contemporary human development, predicting and understanding adult behavior, and explaining how changes in the early development of our ancestors produced contemporary *Homo sapiens*.

Keywords: childhood, evolutionary developmental psychology, developmental systems theory, neoteny, plasticity

ISBNs: 9781108791502 (PB), 9781108866187 (OC)
ISSNs: 2632-9948 (online), 2632-993X (print)

Contents

1 Introduction

"Nothing in biology makes sense except in the light of evolution." So wrote the biologist Theodosius Dobzhansky, reflecting the central role of Darwin's theory of evolution by natural selection for understanding life. This is as true today as it was when Dobzhansky wrote it in 1973. More recently, an appreciation of the centrality of evolutionary theory to the life sciences has extended to psychology, with an increasing number of scholars recognizing the importance of our phylogenetic past for understanding contemporary thought and behavior and how a hairless ape came to be the dominant species of the planet. Some of the last psychologists to join the evolutionary bandwagon were child and developmental scientists, who viewed evolutionary explanations as reflecting *genetic determinism* – genes, evolved over millions of years, determining behavior – leaving little room for the role of culture or experience in general. This misconception has been roundly refuted, and evolutionary perspectives on development have become increasingly accepted to the point where some scholars feel confident saying that "Nothing in *development* makes sense except in the light of evolution" (e.g., Bjorklund & Ellis, 2014; Konner, 2010). An evolutionary perspective can serve as a *metatheory* for development – an overarching set of principles and assumptions to guide research and theory, organize known facts parsimoniously, provide guidance to important domains, and unify the study of development with the rest of the life sciences (Bjorklund, 2018).

In this Element, I present the field of *evolutionary developmental psychology*, defined as "the study of the genetic and ecological mechanisms that govern the development of social and cognitive competencies common to all human beings and the epigenetic (gene-environment interactions) processes that adapt these competencies to local conditions" (Geary & Bjorklund, 2000, p. 57). Evolutionary developmental scientists view development as a natural consequence of species-typical behavior emerging in a species-typical environment that evolved to solve problems associated with survival. Evolutionary developmental science assumes that natural selection has operated as potently (or likely more so) on infants and children as on adults (Bjorklund & Pellegrini, 2002). Before getting to adulthood, individuals had to survive the pre-reproductive stages of life, and natural selection surely influenced these stages as much, or more so, as adulthood. Infancy and childhood can be thought of as the *crucible of natural selection*, with benefits that fostered survival during these stages being selected and maintained for a species (Volk & Atkinson, 2013).

There are two core questions that evolutionary developmental science addresses: (1) How can an understanding of our species' evolution help us better understand children, development, and the adults we become? (2) How can an understanding of human development help us better understand human evolution? In the pages that follow I tackle each of these questions.

2 How Can an Understanding of our Species' Evolution Help Us Better Understand Children, Development, and the Adults We Become?

An evolutionary developmental perspective proposes that children are born with skeletal cognitive mechanisms, shaped by a long history of natural selection, that become fleshed out with experience. These mechanisms are probabilistic in nature and get expressed in a species-typical way only when children experience a species-typical environment. Furthermore, children also possess sufficient plasticity to be sensitive to environmental conditions and adjust their development in anticipation of future environments.

Central to evolutionary psychological theory is the concept of *evolved psychological mechanisms*, domain-specific psychological mechanisms (called *modules*) designed by natural selection to solve specific problems. This metaphor does not lend itself easily to developmental analysis. From this perspective, inherited modules evolved to solve specific problems and are activated under appropriate environmental contexts. They can be thought of as being innate, or perhaps as instincts, with development playing no important role in their expression. There are problems, however, with the concepts of innateness and instincts, in that they are rarely well defined and can have different meaning to different people. This problem was expressed by Bateson (2002, p. 2212) in analyzing the concept "instinct":

> Apart from its colloquial uses, the term instinct has at least nine scientific meanings: present at birth (or at a particular stage of development), not learned, developed before it can be used, unchanged once developed, shared by all members of the species (or at least of the same sex and age), organized into a distinct behavioral system (such as foraging), served by a distinct neural module, adapted during evolution, and differences among individuals that are due to their possession of different genes. One does not necessarily imply another even though people often assume, without evidence, that it does.

Geary (1995, 2005) formulated a model of evolved psychological mechanisms in which development plays a central role and avoids the concept of innateness. Geary conceptualized the human mind as being a set of hierarchically organized information-processing mechanisms, as shown in Figure 1. Geary proposed two overarching domains, one dealing with social information (folk psychology) and the other dealing with ecological information. Each of

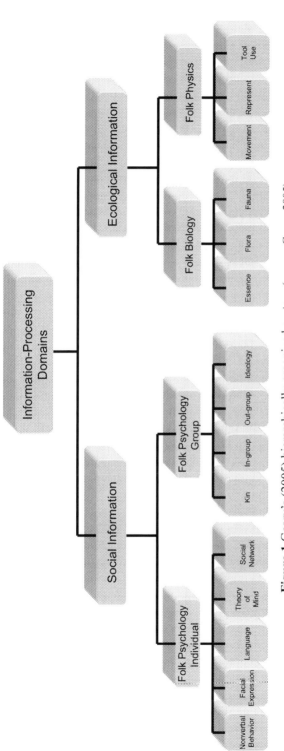

Figure 1 Geary's (2005) hierarchically organized system (source: Geary, 2005).

these domains, in turn, consists of more specific domains (the self, individual, and group for social; biological and physical for ecological), which themselves consist of even more rudimentary domains. From this perspective, information processed at lower levels can be integrated, with complex skills and cognitions emerging through experience.

According to Geary, infants are born with *skeletal competencies* in these various domains, which get fleshed out over development through exploration, play, and social interaction. These skeletal abilities develop in the young of modern humans, developed in the young of our ancestors, and set the stage for the thought and behavior of adults.

Within each domain Geary further distinguished *biologically primary* and *biologically secondary abilities*. Biologically primary abilities were selected by natural selection over the course of evolution. These abilities are species universal and are acquired by children in all but the most deprived environments; children are intrinsically motived to exercise them, with most attaining "expert" level of proficiency. Language is a prototypical type of a biologically primary ability. In contrast, biologically secondary abilities are built on primary abilities, but are cultural inventions. They are not the direct products of natural selection but are determined by each society, and tedious repetition and external pressure are often necessary for their mastery. Biologically secondary abilities could be thought of as *culturally primary abilities*, with reading being a prototypical example.

Geary's acknowledgment of biologically secondary abilities – that have not themselves experienced ancient selection pressures – assumes that humans evolved not simply domain-specific modules to deal with recurrent problems faced by our ancestors, but cognitive mechanisms that are able to adapt to novel circumstances, unanticipated by natural selection (cf., Bornstein & Putnick, 2019). Biologically secondary abilities require neural, cognitive, and behavioral *plasticity* – the ability to change – and a developmental model to explain how inherited information-processing mechanisms become expressed in adults – in some cases to solve recurrent problems faced by our ancestors, but in other cases to solve problems that natural selection could not have anticipated. Evolutionary developmental scientists have adopted variations of *developmental systems theory* to do just that.

2.1 Developmental Systems Theory and the Role of Plasticity in Evolution and Development

Developmental systems theory represents a contemporary approach to the nature-nurture issue – how genes/biology interact with experience/environment to produce behavior. All serious scientists today are transactionists, believing that genes and environment transact over time to produce adult phenotypes. The developmental systems approach provides a particular perspective of how such transactions are accomplished, proposing that development progresses as a continuous, *bidirectional* interaction between components at all levels of the developmental system, including the genetic, cellular, behavioral, ecological, and cultural (e.g., genes ↔ structure ↔ activity ↔ environment; see e.g., Bornstein, 2009; Gottlieb, 2007; West-Eberhard, 2003). At the core of developmental systems theory is the concept of *probabilistic epigenesis*: "individual development is characterized by an increase in novelty and complexity of organization over time – the sequential emergence of new structural and functional properties and competencies – at all levels of analysis as a consequence of horizontal and vertical coactions among its parts, including organism-environment coactions" (Gottlieb, Wahlsten, & Lickliter, 2006, p. 211).

Although genes are a critical component of developmental systems, they are not granted a privileged role in determining behavior but are viewed as one integral part of the system that interacts with other system components. From this perspective genes are not viewed as providing instructions for building a body or generating behavior; rather genes are sensitive to the context in which they find themselves and are influenced by other components of the developmental system. Stated somewhat differently, genes are always expressed in a context, and one cannot partition the effects of genes from those of the environment; the transaction of genes and environment over time together contribute to the emergence of morphology and behavior (see Goldhaber, 2012; Lewkowicz, 2011).[1]

2.1.1 Developmental Systems Theory Provides an Alternative Explanation of "Instinct"

A developmental systems analysis of psychological functioning illustrates that even behaviors usually described as "hard wired" or "innate" require

---

[1] There is no single developmental systems theory, and there is often vigorous debate among theorists about how the theory should be applied. Two broadly defined versions of the theory can be formulated: a soft and a hard version (Bjorklund & Ellis, 2014; Del Giudice & Ellis, 2016). The soft version is essentially a theory of development in which a developmental system comprises all the "resources" (genes, cellular structures, sensory experiences, physical parameters of the environment, and so forth) that contribute to the development of the individual organism. Development proceeds via the continuous bidirectional interaction between the organism and the environment, but the organism is the focus of natural selection, as in mainstream biology. In contrast, in the hard version of developmental systems theory, the entire organism-environment whole of replicable developmental systems is the focus of natural selection. This removes the organism as the focus of natural selection, and natural selection can only operate at the population level (see Overton, 2015; Witherington & Lickliter, 2016). The hard form of developmental systems theory is incompatible with an adaptationist perspective, and it is the soft form of developmental systems theory that evolutionary developmental scientists advocate (see Bjorklund, 2016).

individuals possessing both species-typical genomes *and* species-typical environments for their proper expression. For example, there is no debate that genes
provide information for the construction of the nervous and perceptual systems
that result, shortly after birth (or sometimes even before), in the experiences of
sensation. The visual cortex, for example, receives input from the optic nerve
producing "sight." Yet, for the visual system to develop properly, the young
organism must have visual input from the eyes. For most members of a species,
development proceeds "as usual," and animals are quickly able to make sense of
their visual world. However, when organisms receive species-atypical, delayed,
or no visual experience at all early in life, the brain and the ability to see develop
in a species-*atypical* way. Such atypical development was illustrated in classic
research with cats and rats. For example, animals raised in total darkness or
exposed only to homogeneous light without seeing any patterns, later have
difficulty making simple visual discriminations (e.g., Crabtree & Riesen, 1979),
as do animals raised so they see only vertical patterns (Hubel & Wiesel, 1962).
Experience (or lack thereof) changes the structure and organization of the young
brain, even for processes as basic as vision. Similar outcomes are also seen in
human infants who are born with cataracts over their eyes, preventing them
from seeing patterned light. Infants who have cataracts removed within the first
2 or 3 months of life develop mostly normal vision, although vision is impaired
when cataracts are not removed until later in development (Le Grand et al.,
2001; Maurer, Mondloch, & Lewis, 2007; see Maurer & Lewis, 2013 for
a review). Such findings reflect the idea of a *critical*, or *sensitive period*,
a time – usually early in development – when certain experiences most significantly impact brain organization and function (such as seeing). The same
experience before or after the sensitive period will have little or no effect on
development (see Bornstein, 1989).

   As another example of how presumably "innate" behavior actually is dependent on experience, consider the phenomenon of imprinting in precocial birds.
The Austrian ethologist and Nobel laureate Konrad Lorenz (1952) demonstrated that goslings and other precocial birds would approach the first moving
and vocalizing object (usually their mother) they encountered several hours
after hatching, forming an attachment to that object. Such *imprinting*, Lorenz
contended, occurred without prior experience, providing a classic demonstration of an instinct. However, hours-old precocial birds are not totally without
experience when tested for imprinting. For example, they have heard the
vocalizations of their mother and brood mates, both in the days before and the
hours after hatching. In a series of carefully controlled experiments, Gottlieb
(1976) manipulated what pre-hatched ducklings heard – the quacking of their
mother, the peeps of their brood mates, and finally – isolating each egg – only

the duckling's own peeps. In each case, newly hatched ducklings approached the maternal call of their own species (e.g., mallard) versus the maternal call of a related species (e.g., wood duck). These results seemed to support Lorenz's contention that auditory imprinting was indeed an instinct, requiring no prior experience for its demonstration. But even the isolated ducklings had some relevant experience – their own peeps – which share auditory features with the species' adult call. Gottlieb developed a surgical technique wherein, days prior to hatching, before the birds begin to vocalize, he placed glue on the birds' vocal cords, preventing them from producing any sounds. (This effect wears off several days after hatching.) Under these conditions, the hatchlings were unable to differentiate the maternal calls of a bird from their own species (e.g., mallard) versus another species (e.g., wood duck). Some experience was necessary for these birds to become imprinted to a conspecific – a type of experience that nearly all ducklings would receive, except perhaps those hatched in Gottlieb's lab.

2.1.2 Developmental Systems Theory and Plasticity

Central to developmental systems theory is the idea that organisms have substantial plasticity, especially early in development. For example, research with precocial birds, such as Gottlieb's ducks, has shown that providing pre-hatchlings with species-atypical experience (e.g., exposure to vocalizations of another species, vestibular stimulation, patterned light) alters aspects of post-hatching perception (e.g., Kenny & Turkewitz, 1986; Lickliter, 1990). For instance, when Lickliter (1990) exposed bobwhite-quail embryos to patterned light days before hatching, the chicks later showed disrupted auditory attach-ment (failing to approach the maternal bobwhite-quail call), but also some enhancements in visual discrimination abilities. Most members of a species turn out to be highly similar to one another because they inherit both a species-typical genome and a species-typical environment. However, when young animals received species-*atypical* experience (e.g., delayed or earlier-than-expected stimulation), species-*atypical* behaviors and abilities develop. Such variable outcomes can only happen when organisms have the plasticity early in life to permit such influences. Animals' developing brains, physiology, and behaviors are coordinated with species-typical experiences, both pre- and postnatally, to reliably produce species-typical behavior (including behaviors that were once called "instincts"). As Bjorklund and Ellis (2005, p. 13) stated, "genetic information is extensively scaffolded by species-typical features of the environment, and the phenotypic outcome is a predictable, emergent property of the total developmental system."

Child Development

2.1.3 Plasticity in Human Development

Plasticity is greatest early in life and decreases with time. Yet, humans are perhaps the most neurologically, cognitively, and behaviorally plastic of all animals, retaining a high degree of plasticity late into life. This extended plasticity is provided by a large and slow-developing brain (relative to other primates). At birth people have nearly all the neurons they will ever have (adults have approximately 86 billion neurons), although these neurons are small in size and have fewer connections with other neurons than they will have as adults. Most neurons in newborns lack *myelin*, the fatty coating that serves to insulate axons resulting in faster and more efficient transmission of nervous signals. Over the next several years, a process of pruning called *apoptosis* or *selective cell death*, occurs, while surviving neurons increase in size, in number of connections with other neurons, and myelination of their axons. Importantly, experience plays a major role in determining these connections. (I will discuss human brain development and evolution in more detail in Section 3.)

There is substantial evidence for high levels of neural plasticity early in life. For example, young children show a remarkable ability to recover from some forms of brain damage. This is clearly apparent in the most-studied types of brain damage, those associated with insults to areas of the brain dealing with language. Evidence has accumulated since the nineteenth century that young children with damage to language areas of the brain show far greater recovery of function than older children or adults (see Witelson, 1987). To quote Witelson (1987, p. 676), "there is a remarkable functional plasticity for language functions following brain damage in childhood in that the eventual cognitive level reached is often far beyond that observed in cases of adult brain damage, even those having extensive remedial education. These results attest to the operation of marked neural plasticity at least in the immature brain." Similar patterns are observed for less-severe brain injuries such as concussions (see Yeats & Taylor, 2005).

Other research has shown that children who encounter deleterious early experience, such as lack of social and physical stimulation as a result of institutionalization, show serious social, emotional, and intellectual deficits, but that those negative effects can be reversed when children's life conditions change for the better (e.g., Beckett et al., 2006; Nelson et al., 2007; Rutter et al., 2007). Children's extended period of brain development affords them the plasticity to radically alter their course of ontogeny in response to changes in their environment. However, such plasticity is not infinite. Children who spend their first two years in socially nonstimulating environments frequently continue to display social, emotional, and cognitive deficits, even when placed in more supportive homes (e.g., Bick et al., 2018; Merz et al., 2016; Nelson et al., 2007). Not surprisingly, extended institutionalization is also associated with changes in brain structure and functioning (e.g., Tottenham et al., 2010).

2.1.4 Epigenetics and Plasticity

It should not be surprising that environmental effects, such as spending one's first two years in a nonstimulating environment, influence the brain. Scientists have long known that the brain is the organ responsible for psychological phenomena, with modern technology allowing researchers to pinpoint where in the brain functioning is affected and how different parts of the brain communicate with one another to produce emotion, cognition, and behavior. What is perhaps more surprising is how experience alters the expression of DNA, which in turn affects psychological changes in the organism. The emerging field of *epigenetics* is helping to explain how, at the molecular level, experience affects behavior, and thus to develop a better understanding of plasticity.

At its most basic, epigenetics refers to how genes are expressed in different contexts (Moore, 2015). Not only do plants and animals inherit genes from their parents, but also chemical markers that regulate the expression of genes. Biologists once believed that epigenetic effects were active only early in development, instructing genes to create specific structures and organs (fingers and toes; lungs and livers, for example), and then turning off those genes once the structures and organs had been formed. Chemicals in the cytoplasm of cells deactivate genes so that one has only 10 toes and 2 lungs, both situated in the proper places in the body. In recent years, biologists have learned that epigenetic processes occur not only in early development but throughout life, and they seem to be the mechanism responsible for modifying genetic activity as a result of experience.

There is a variety of biochemical processes involved in epigenetics, with *DNA methylation* being the most studied and best understood. Chemicals from the methyl group (written CH_3 by chemists) found in the cytoplasm of cells can become attached to some of the nucleic acids (the chemical components of DNA), which alter what a particular stretch of DNA "does." Structural genes provide instructions for the formation of proteins, and genes that are highly methylated shut down their production. Other cytoplasmic chemicals can become attached to stretches of DNA effectively activating genes, a process called *acetylation*.

DNA methylation can be measured through blood or scrapings from the inside of a person's cheek. Methylation, or other epigenetic processes, is the primary mechanism by which experience modifies gene action and thus behavior. For instance, some research has identified epigenetic markers associated with early adverse environments and subsequent chronic aggression (Trembly & Szyf, 2010). In one study, 11- to 14-year-old children who had been mal-treated displayed greater methylation to a gene associated with stress regulation and to a gene associated with nerve growth factor than nonmaltreated children (Romens et al., 2015). Other research using saliva (Parades et al., 2016) or placental blood (Kertes et al., 2016) has shown that early stress is related to the methylation of genes associated with the expression of the stress hormone cortisol and to subsequent internalizing behavior. Pregnant women's ratings of hardship during the 1998 Quebec Ice Storm were related to levels of DNA methylation in their children's genes associated with the immune system 13 years later (Cao-Lei et al., 2014). Findings such as these are consistent with the argument made by van IJzendoorn and his colleagues (2011) that child devel-opment can be defined as "experiences being sculpted in the organism's DNA through methylation" (p. 305).

Behavioral epigenetics is in its infancy but holds great promise for under-standing how experience changes the behavior of an organism and of the very process of plasticity itself. Some researchers have emphasized the insights epigenetic mechanisms can play in our understanding, specifically with respect to the development of mental health associated with early-life stress (e.g., Melas et al., 2013). To quote Conradt (2017, p. 111), "epigenetic research can advance research on early-life stress because epigenetic processes may help explain how early-life stress becomes biologically embedded and which children are most susceptible to this stress." Epigenetics also has important implications for how species change over evolutionary time, and I will briefly revisit the role epigen-etics might have played in human phylogeny in Section 3.

2.2 Evolved Probabilistic Cognitive Mechanisms

Children have been prepared through natural selection to process some infor-mation more effectively than others (e.g., language, some social relations), but they are constrained both by their biology and their physical and social envir-onments in how they make sense of their world. *But prepared is not preformed* (Bjorklund, 2003). Instead of viewing psychological mechanisms as innate, they can be seen as originating from low-level cognitive and perceptual abil-ities, or cognitive primitives, that develop into adaptive behavior and thought when children experience a species-typical environment. Such mechanisms are not preformed, executed when triggered by an appropriate stimulus, but rather develop through Gene x Environment x Development interactions that emerge in each generation, are influenced by prenatal as well as postnatal environments, and reflect the inheritance of developmental systems, not just genes (see Coen, 2000). To capture this idea, my colleagues and I proposed the concept of *evolved probabilistic cognitive mechanisms*, defined as:

> information-processing mechanisms that have evolved to solve recurrent problems faced by ancestral populations; however, they are expressed in a probabilistic fashion in each individual in a generation, based on the continuous and bidirectional interaction over time at all levels of organization, from the genetic through the cultural. These mechanisms are universal, in that they will develop in a species-typical manner when an individual experiences a species-typical environment over the course of ontogeny (Bjorklund, Ellis, & Rosenberg, 2007, p. 22).

Children do not inherit "instincts" or mental operations that are "ready to go" when exposed to a particular context. Rather, what is inherited are perceptual/ cognitive/behavioral biases that, in interaction with a child's environment, produce a pattern of (usually) adaptive thinking or behavior. Children's neurological maturation is coordinated with species-typical experiences, such that most members of a species, be they bobwhite quail, chimpanzees, or humans, develop to be much like one another. Yet, the high level of neural plasticity, especially in *Homo sapiens* infants and youth, means that developmental outcomes are not predetermined but can differ as a result of variations in early experiences. Children evolved to be sensitive to features of early environments and to adjust their developmental trajectory accordingly. Evolved probabilistic cognitive mechanisms are not instincts as they are typically conceived, but rather emerge from initial perceptual and information-processing biases in interaction with species-typical environments.

As an example of evolved probabilistic cognitive mechanisms, consider humans' fear of snakes. Although fear of snakes seems to be universal (with many individual differences), infants are not born fearful of snakes, but rather, much as adults (Öhman, Flykt, & Esteves, 2001), are especially attentive to snakes, and, much as monkeys (Cook & Mineka, 1989), can easily acquire an aversion to them when moving images of snakes are associated with negative affect (see DeLoache & LoBue, 2009; LoBue & Adolph, 2019). Apparently, it is snakes' unique sinusoidal movement, distinct from the movement of mammals, that attracts infants' attention and was used by natural selection to help children develop a fear of this prehistorically dangerous class of animals.

One highly important social stimulus in an infant's world is faces (particularly the face of one's mother). Newborns, in fact, have a number of perceptual biases that attract them to faces, as well as mechanisms that make the processing of face-like stimuli more efficient than other stimuli. For instance, newborns tend to look at face-like stimuli (e.g., Mondloch et al., 1999); are especially attentive to faces with eyes open and gazing at them (e.g., Farroni et al., 2002);

spend more time looking at their mothers' faces than at faces of other women (e.g., Bushnell, Sai, & Mullin, 1989); look longer at right-side-up versus inverted faces, but only when they can see the eyes (Gava et al., 2008); and discriminate between human and nonhuman faces (e.g., Sanefuji et al., 2014). Neonates do not necessarily understand the social meaning of faces, but instead are attentive to certain perceptual features that characterize faces, including movement (Haith, 1966) and areas of high contrast, such as eyes (Salapatek & Kessen, 1966). Over the next several months, as a result of neurological maturation and experience, infants show biases to attend to curvilinear stimuli (Ruff & Birch, 1974), vertically symmetrical stimuli (i.e., the right and left sides of a stimulus are symmetrical) (e.g., Griffey & Little, 2014), and have biases to attend to "top-heavy" stimuli (i.e., up-down asymmetry), with this bias being found even in newborns (Macchi Cassia, Turati, & Simion, 2004). By 3 months of age, infants can discriminate among faces of different species, sexes, and races equally well, but with increasing experience their perceptual ability narrows, so that by 9 months infants are increasingly able to discriminate among faces they see frequently (e.g., women, their own race) but less able to discriminate among faces from other species (Pascalis et al., 2002), races (Kelly, Liu et al., 2009), or men (Quinn et al., 2002). Such adaptations are not inevitable and will not emerge if children experience a species-atypical environment (e.g., frequently seeing monkey faces [Pascalis et al., 2005], faces from other races [Anzures et al., 2012], or their fathers are their primary caregivers [Quinn et al., 2002]).

Although young infants are attentive to faces and seem to process faces especially effectively, it is not faces per se they are attentive to, but rather a suite of low-level perceptual features that faces happen to possess (movement, curvilinearity, top-heavy asymmetry), coupled with some processing biases (being able to discriminate among top-heavy stimuli better than horizontally symmetrical or bottom-heavy stimuli) that provide faces with their privileged processing status. With maturation and experience, infants' face-processing abilities improve, but selectively, for classes of faces they experience most frequently. Yet, infants retain enough plasticity that developmental trajectories can be modified, permitting Caucasian infants, for example, to maintain (or regain) their ability to differentiate between faces from a different race or even a different species.

2.3 Adaptations of Infancy and Childhood

Adaptation is a key concept in evolutionary psychology and biology. Buss and his colleagues (1998, p. 535) defined an adaptation as "an inherited and reliably developing characteristic that came into existence as a feature of a species through natural selection because it helped to directly or indirectly facilitate reproduction during the period of its evolution." Consistent with the concept of evolved probabilistic cognitive mechanisms, adaptations arise from reliable Genes x Environment x Development interactions; thus, adaptations have both an evolutionary and a developmental history (Bjorklund, 2015; Hernández Blasi & Bjorklund, 2003).

Although some adaptations may be useful throughout life, others may be especially important, or take a slightly different form, during infancy and childhood. Evolutionary developmental scientists distinguish different types of childhood adaptations: *ontogenetic adaptations* adapt infants and children to their immediate environment and not necessarily to a future one (Bjorklund, 1997). They serve to help the young organism adjust to the current ecological niche and not necessarily to a future adult life. In contrast, *deferred adaptations* were selected, at least in part, for their role in preparing children for adulthood (Hernández Blasi & Bjorklund, 2003). They may also serve an immediate benefit to the children who possess them, but they continue to be useful in later life. For example, many social-cognitive processes dedicated to cooperating and competing with peers are useful during childhood and in many cases may serve to prepare children for similar interactions during adulthood. In the next sections I provide some examples of both ontogenetic and deferred adaptations.

2.3.1 Ontogenetic Adaptations

Perhaps the clearest examples of ontogenetic adaptations come from prenatal development. For example, mammals receive nutrients and rid themselves of waste products through the umbilical cord and placenta. Once born, these organs and the physiological mechanisms associated with them are discarded as the newborn's respiratory and consummatory systems become reorganized. The adaptations served to keep the individual alive at a specific time in development, in this case during the prenatal period. Similar behavioral and psychological adaptations can be identified after birth, adapting children to the niche of childhood.

One candidate for an ontogenetic adaptation during early infancy is *neonatal imitation*, in which infants over the first two months of life will (sometimes) match the facial expression modeled by an adult (e.g., sticking out their tongues or pursing their lips; Meltzoff & Moore, 1977). Babies often fail to make the same facial gesture they saw a model make, but instead will make *some* facial response (e.g., sticking out their tongues even when they saw a model purse her lips) greater than expected by chance (Oostenbroek et al., 2016; Redshaw et al., 2019).

Initial interpretations of neonatal imitation suggested that it reflected sophisticated social learning from birth; more recent interpretations have proposed that
neonatal imitation is best viewed as an ontogenetic adaptation, designed to
promote infant-mother interaction during a time when infants are unable to
intentionally control their own behavior (Bjorklund, 1987, 2018; Byrne, 2005;
Nagy, 2006), then disappearing when more sophisticated social-cognitive abilities develop to control social interaction. This interpretation is supported by the
fact that neonatal imitation disappears around two months of age when higher-
cortical brain areas are able to influence infants' intentional actions (see Periss &
Bjorklund, 2011) and by research reporting that infants who showed high levels
of imitation at birth had better quality social interactions with their mothers three
months later than infants with low levels of neonatal imitation (Heimann, 1989;
see also Simpson et al., 2016, for evidence with monkeys).

Another candidate for an ontogenetic adaptation of infancy and early childhood is the *baby schema* (*kindschenschema*; Lorenz, 1943). The baby schema
includes chubby cheeks, flat nose, rounded and large head relative to body size,
large eyes, and short and broad extremities. For instance, adults view infants
whose features more closely match the prototypical baby schema as cuter than
babies with fewer baby-schema features and (1) rate them more positively on
attributes such as warmth and honesty (e.g., Senese et al., 2013); (2) express
greater motivation for caregiving (e.g., Glocker et al., 2009); (3) show more
affectionate interactions toward (Langlois et al., 1995); (4) express greater
empathy for (Machluf & Bjorklund, 2016); and (5) make hypothetical adoption
decisions about (Waller, Volk, & Quinsey, 2004), than less-cute infants (see
Franklin & Volk, 2018; Kringelbach et al., 2016; and Lucion et al., 2017 for
reviews). Other research has shown that children with cuter, more attractive
faces continue to elicit positive responses from adults until approximately
4.5 years of age, after which ratings of likability and attractiveness of children's
faces are similar to ratings of adult faces (Luo, Li, & Lee, 2011). However,
adults are especially sensitive to other cues of immaturity in evaluating older
preschool-age children. These include voices (children with more immature
voices are rated as more likable, cuter, friendlier, nicer, and helpless than
children with more mature voices, Hernández Blasi et al., 2018), and some
expressions of immature cognition (e.g., "The sun's not out because it's mad,"
Hernández Blasi et al., 2015), suggesting that some ontogenetic adaptations are
found past infancy into childhood.

One example of an ontogenetic adaptation of childhood is children's
unrealistic optimism regarding their own abilities. Preschool and early school-
age children tend to greatly overestimate their abilities and their positive traits,
believing they are stronger, smarter, more popular, more attractive, have better

memories, and have better physical abilities than objective evaluations would warrant (e.g., Boulton & Smith, 1990; Stipek, 1981; Schneider, 1998). Children's overly positive assessments are not due to poor cognition in general; they are typically more accurate judging the abilities and traits of other children. It is mainly for themselves they reserve the overly optimistic evaluations (Stipek, 1981).

How might such unrealistic optimism be adaptive to young children? Bandura (1997) proposed that people with high levels of *self-efficacy* perceive themselves to be in control of specific aspects of their lives and behave accordingly. Young children have been described as universal novices, and as such they rarely excel at any of the tasks they attempt. By having an overly positive assessment of their own performance and talents, children may persist at tasks where a person with a more accurate assessment of their abilities (or inabilities) might quit. Their immature cognition may protect them from perceiving failure and damaging their sense of self-efficacy. Consistent with this argument, young children who overestimate their task performance (e.g., how many words they will remember; how well they imitated a model) actually show higher levels of performance (or faster improvement on a task) than more accurate children (e.g., Bjorklund, Gaultney, & Green, 1993; Shin, Bjorklund, & Beck, 2007). Children become more accurate in assessing their own abilities by middle childhood (Stipek, 1984), and children who are better at assessing their abilities tend to show a cognitive advantage (see Schneider, 1985), a reversal of what is found for younger children. Young children also believe that psychological and physical traits tend to improve over time and that people have substantial control in changing traits, a phenomenon called *protective optimism* (Lockhart, Chang, & Tyler, 2002; Lockhart, Goddu, & Keil, 2017).

Seligmann (1991) captured well young children's unrealistic opinions of themselves, proposing that young children's extreme optimism was selected in human evolution: "The child carries the seed of the future, and nature's primary interest in children is that they reach puberty safely and produce the next generation of children. Nature has buffered our children not only physically – prepubescent children have the lowest death rate from all causes – but psychologically as well, by endowing them with hope, abundant and irrational" (p. 126). We do not totally lose an unrealistic evaluation of ourselves as we age. For example, adults consistently believe they are more skilled and better-than-average at most things than an objective assessment would indicate (e.g., Shepperd et al., 2013; Zell et al., 2020). However, few well-functioning adults display such a positive opinion of themselves as the average 4- or 5-year-old.

2.3.2 Deferred Adaptations

If you asked most people, including developmental scientists, what childhood was *for*, the most common short answer would be preparation for adulthood. This must be true to a certain extent, as the many things children learn on their journey to adulthood are skills and knowledge that will be useful in their lives as grown-ups. Yet, we have seen that some adaptations are important only during a certain time in development and disappear (or change substantially) as children age. Moreover, natural selection does not have a crystal ball, but rather adapts individuals to current local environments, not future ones. How, then, can some adaptations of infancy and childhood be deferred, providing benefits to environments that the organism has yet to experience?

The answer to this question is that adaptations that prepare children for life in adulthood also have some *immediate* benefits. For example, play, which I discuss in more detail shortly, not only fosters social-cognitive skills that will be useful to people when navigating adult social hierarchies, but also benefits children while they play. Children as well as adults glean benefits from successful social inter-actions – identifying in-group from out-group members, learning from observing others, and collaborating to achieve difficult goals. (I will discuss the development of some of these social-cognitive abilities later in this section.) With this in mind I turn to perhaps the most ubiquitous of deferred adaptations, children's play.

Play

Play is the quintessential activity of childhood. It's what children in all cultures *do*. In fact, the ubiquity of play may cause people to overlook its significance. Counter to popular opinion, play is not just something children do until they gain the physical, social, and cognitive abilities for more serious endeavors, such as work or formal schooling. Yet, the very definition of play can give the impression of frivolousness. Play is something organisms engage in voluntarily and for its own sake. Play is not done with the intent to learn, to acquire resources, or to improve one's social standing. Although any or all of these things may be gained through play, that is not its intention. Play is, by definition, purposeless; it is its own reward. Yet, scholars have long recognized that youthful play is essential for proper development and the acquisition of import-ant knowledge and skills. To quote an early play researcher, "animals cannot be said to play because they are young and frolicsome, *but rather they have a period of youth in order to play*" (Groos, 1898/1975, p. 75). This is no less true of human children as it is of nonhuman animals.

Play comes in a variety of forms. *Locomotive play* involves running, chasing (or being chased), climbing, wrestling, and play fighting (the latter two referred to as *rough-and-tumble play*), each of which fosters coordination, physical development, learning about the local environment, and, when done with other children, learning about social interaction, including skills that might be useful in adulthood (see Bjorklund & Pellegrini, 2002, and Pellegrini & Smith, 1998 for reviews). *Object play* involves manipulating objects, which helps children learn about the qualities or properties of objects (i.e., their *affordances*) and may be important in learning about human artifacts and tools (Pellegrini, 2013a). For example, Smith (1982) proposed that object play prepares children to use tools "over and above what could be learnt through observation, imitation, and goal-directed practice." Similarly, Lockman (2000, p. 137) stated that "the origins of tool use in humans can be found during much of the first year of life, in the perception-action routines that infants repeatedly display as they explore their environments."

Locomotive and object play are found in all social mammals, but *fantasy play*, or make-believe, seems to be unique to humans. (But see Gómez & Martín-Andrade, 2005, for a suggestion that some rudimentary forms of fantasy play are displayed by enculturated, or human-reared, apes.) Fantasy play involves children engaging in *counterfactual thinking*, taking an "as if" perspective by representing objects and people in a form other than what they really are, something Nielsen (2012) proposed was necessary for the evolution of human intelligence. Counterfactual thinking is most easily seen during *socio-dramatic play*, which is first observed around three years of age, with children taking on imaginary roles and staying "in character" throughout the play bout, being fully aware that what they are doing is not "real" (e.g., Lillard et al., 2013). Children may play at being superheroes (truly fantasy characters), people engaging in everyday activities that they observe in their culture (such as "mommies and daddies" or "teachers and students"), or wished-for adult roles, such as astronauts or firefighters. In traditional cultures, sociodramatic play often involves adult survival tasks, such as hunting or cooking (e.g., Bock & Johnson, 2004).

Play seems to be the principal mechanism by which children in traditional cultures learn the skills necessary for adult functioning. Although teaching seems to be the primary mechanism by which children in developed societies[2] acquire important cultural skills (first from their parents and later from

---

[2] Most psychological research has been done in developed societies, or what have been called WEIRD (Western, Educated, Industrial, Rich, Democratic) cultures (Henrich et al., 2010; Nielsen et al., 2017). It has become increasingly obvious that generalizing findings from research performed in WEIRD cultures to all of humanity is highly problematic, and this is especially true when taking an evolutionary perspective. WEIRD societies do not reflect the conditions in which human psychology evolved. For this reason, whenever possible, research performed in non-WEIRD cultures is reported when available.

teachers), this is not the case in traditional cultures. Adults in traditional cultures rarely explicitly engage in teaching children. In fact, when teaching occurs in hunter-gatherer cultures, particularly in the realm of foraging, children rather than adults are more apt to play the role of teacher (Lew-Levy et al., 2020). Hunter-gatherer children learn mainly through observing others (social learning) and through play in mixed-age groups (Gray, 2016; Lancy, 2015). However, play continues to be an important mechanism of learning for children in developed societies, especially social skills, and children's play has also been shown to be positively related to cognitive functioning. For example, the more time 3-year-olds spent talking with peers during fantasy play the larger their vocabularies were two years later (Elias & Berk, 2002). Other research has found similar positive relations between the amount of spontaneous sociodramatic play children engage in and their subsequent memory for and comprehension of stories (e.g., Pellegrini & Galda, 1982; Smilansky, 1968). The amount of time children spend in free play is positively related to levels of *executive function* (e.g., Barker et al., 2014; Carlson, White, & Davis-Unger, 2014; Elias & Berk, 2002). Executive function includes working memory, inhibition, and cognitive flexibility (e.g., Garon, Bryson, & Smith, 2008; McAuley & White, 2011) and is a central component to planning and the performance of many higher-order cognitive abilities, including reading, mathematics, theory of mind, and general intelligence, among others (see Bjorklund & Causey, 2018 for a review).

The play of boys and girls tends to differ in predictable ways across cultures, and these sex differences are good candidates for deferred adaptations. For example, perhaps the most obvious sex difference in play style is for rough-and-tumble play. Boys engage in more rough-and-tumble play than girls, which some authorities have proposed prepares boys for intrasexual competition (see Geary 2021; Pellegrini & Smith, 1998). Such play may be especially important for boys in hunter-gatherer societies, preparing them for hunting and warfare at the group level (Keeley, 1996). Similar sex differences in rough-and-tumble play have been found in other social mammals (e.g., Smith, 1982).

With respect to object play, boys are also more likely to engage in play with objects than girls (e.g., Bornstein et al., 1996; Caldera et al., 1989; see Pellegrini, 2013a). One study reported that 3-year-old boys engaged in more object-oriented play than 3-year-old girls and outperformed girls on a subsequent lure-retrieval task in which children had to select and use the proper tool to retrieve a desired toy. Moreover, whereas the amount of object play predicted how well boys would do on the lure-retrieval task, the relation between object play and task performance was not significant for girls (Gredlein & Bjorklund, 2005). The authors suggested that "boys may be more sensitive to such environmental experiences [afforded by object play] than girls, and that some gender-related factors (e.g., prenatal hormone exposure) other than amount of object play contribute significantly to the observed differences in tool use" (Gredlein & Bjorklund, 2005, p. 227). These findings are consistent with Geary's (2005, 2021) argument discussed earlier that infants possess a small set of skeletal competencies specialized to process information relating to their social, biological, and physical worlds that get fleshed out with experience, here experience playing with objects. Geary proposed that sex differences in early behavior interact with these still-developing skeletal competencies, resulting in different outcomes for boys and girls, and that young boys may be especially sensitive to actions on objects, benefiting more from object play than girls (Geary, 2021).

Finally, although both boys and girls engage in fantasy play, the themes of their play tend to be quite different, and this is true across a wide range of cultures. Girls' fantasy play tends to emphasize relationships and domestic themes (e.g., playing house, school), whereas the fantasy play of boys is more focused on dominance themes (e.g., superheroes versus supervillains, cops and robbers; Pellegrini, 2013b). Such play may have prepared ancestral boys and girls for the lives they would likely experience as adults, with women's relationships being more intimate and men's relationships more based on status.

The deferred benefits of play include the skills and knowledge children acquire during play, which can serve as the foundation for skills in later life. The amount of free play children engage in predicts aspects of adult socio-emotional functioning: Children who engaged in greater amounts of free play grew up to have higher self-esteem, better friendships, and better general psychological and physical health (Greve & Thomsen, 2016; Greve, Thomsen, & Dehio, 2014). The researchers reported that the benefits in adulthood of childhood free play were mediated by greater adaptivity (flexible goal adjustment).

Conditional Adaptations and Life History Theory

Conditional adaptations are a type of deferred adaptation in which children's sensitivity to their current environment causes them to adjust aspects of their development in anticipation of future circumstances. Boyce and Ellis (2005, p. 290) defined conditional adaptations as "evolved mechanisms that detect and respond to specific features of childhood environments – features that have proven reliable over evolutionary time in predicting the nature of the social and physical world into which children will mature – and entrain developmental pathways that reliably matched those features during a species' natural selective history." Children evolved a high level of behavioral, cognitive, and neural plasticity, permitting them to modify aspects of their ontogeny to match current and anticipated environments (e.g., Belsky et al., 1991). Conditional adaptations are what underlie children's abilities to adapt their developmental paths as a function of the local ecology's levels of harshness and predictability in anticipation of the quality of future environments, and is likely best reflected by contemporary research in life history theory.

Life history theory has its origins in behavioral ecology (see Del Giudice, Gangestad, & Kaplan, 2016; Hill & Kaplan, 1999; Stearns, 1992) and examines decisions animals make in allocating time and energy to various aspects of their development. How much time and energy should individuals invest in mating versus parenting, somatic growth versus reproduction, current development (or reproduction) versus later development (or reproduction)? How individuals respond to these trade-offs constitutes their *life history strategy*, which exists on a continuum from fast to slow (see Figure 2). A *fast life history strategy* is characteristic of short-lived animals (high mortality) or animals living in harsh and unpredictable environments. Under these conditions, it is adaptive to take risks, to mature and reproduce quickly, invest little in long-term relationships, have many offspring, and adopt an opportunistic

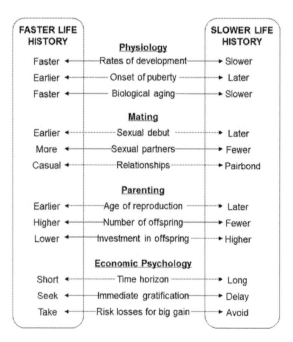

Figure 2 The fast-slow continuum of life history variation
(source: Ellis et al., 2012).

versus a futuristic orientation. In contrast, a *slow life history strategy* is typical of long-lived animals (low mortality) or animals living in environments with plentiful resources (nonharsh), high predictability, and reliable relationships. Under these conditions it makes sense to develop more slowly (put more resources into developing one's body and behavioral skills), avoid risk, invest more in relationships and in a small number of children, and plan for the future.

Evolutionarily minded developmental scientists have proposed that life history theory can be applied to individuals within a species and that children are highly sensitive to early environmental conditions, especially those related to harshness and predictability, and adjust important aspects of their developmental trajectory in anticipation of future environments. Belsky, Steinberg, and Draper (1991) specifically applied life history theory to human development:

> a principal evolutionary function of early experience – the first 5–7 years of life – is to induce in the child an understanding of the availability and predictability of resources (broadly defined) in the environment, of the trustworthiness of others, and of the enduringness of close interpersonal relationships, all of which will affect how the developing person apportions reproductive effort (p. 650).

According to Belsky and his colleagues, children evolved the neural and behavioral plasticity necessary to adjust important aspects of their development to match current and anticipated environments. Subsequent research has shown that harshness and/or predictability of children's early home environments is related to the onset and frequency of risk-taking, sexual activity, incidence of teenage pregnancy, and antisocial behavior in adolescents or young adults (e.g., Chang et al., 2019; Ellis et al., 2009; Simpson et al., 2012; Szepsenwol et al., 2018; for evidence that early-life adversity accelerates child and adolescent development generally, see Belsky, 2019).

Consider, for example, research by Simpson and his colleagues (2012) that examined the relation between children's early life experiences and subsequent behavior at age 23. Children growing up in highly unpredictable environments during their first five years – reflected by changes in residences, parental job changes, and different adult males living in the household – had their first sexual encounter earlier, had more sex partners, and engaged in higher levels of risk-taking and delinquent behaviors than children growing up in more predictable homes. The quality of children's home environment from age 6 to 16 was *not* related to later behavior, indicating it was experience during the preschool years that was primarily responsible for shaping later behavior.

Psychologists generally see harsh and unpredictable environments as producing only negative consequences – disrupting normal development and adversely affecting children's well-being. However, from an evolutionary developmental perspective, early stressful environments do not so much disrupt development as they direct it toward strategies that are adaptive (or were for our ancestors) under harsh conditions. Although the behaviors of adolescents and adults following a fast life history strategy may be socially problematic and maladaptive from the perspective of middle-class society, they may be adaptive from an evolutionary perspective. An opportunistic lifestyle provides some potentially adaptive outcomes for children growing up in harsh and unpredictable circumstances (Ellis et al., 2009, 2012). Moreover, children following a fast life history strategy in response to harsh and unpredictable environments may possess "hidden talents," enhanced cognitive and social abilities adapted to stressful or unpredictable conditions (e.g., Ellis et al., 2017; Frankenhuis et al., 2019). For example, Mittal and his colleagues (2015) reported that children who experienced harsh and unpredictable early environments would later, as adults, display deficits in inhibition but were better at task shifting compared to people who experienced less-harsh and more stable early environments. The authors proposed that inhibition can be disadvantageous when ecological conditions favor opportunism, whereas the ability to shift effectively between contexts is critical for adapting to unpredictable environments. Succeeding in harsh and uncertain environments likely requires prioritizing short-term success over what is best in the long-term, allowing for the selection of these adaptations.

Differential Susceptibility to Environmental Influence

Although life history theory can account for some of the differences observed for children growing up in "easy" versus "difficult" environments, much variability in behavioral and cognitive outcomes is left unexplained. Different children from the same neighborhood or the same family do not always show the same developmental pattern. Rather, some children are more sensitive to the effects of harshness and predictability than others, and such individual differences are captured by the concept of *differential susceptibility to environmental influence*, which proposes that children (and adults) are differentially sensitive to the effects of their environments (e.g., Belsky & Pluess, 2009; Ellis, Boyce, et al., 2011). At one extreme are children who have especially high levels of plasticity, which makes them more susceptible to the effects of both extremely positive and negative environments. These are sometimes referred to as *orchid children*, who, like orchids, flourish under supportive conditions but fare poorly in neglectful ones. At the other extreme are *dandelion children*, who, like the flower (or the weed), survive in nearly all environments. Dandelion children may do slightly better under more supportive than less supportive circumstances, but they are not especially sensitive to a range of both positive and negative environments, doing well under most conditions. The orchid-dandelion distinction is actually a continuum, with about 20 percent of children displaying high levels of biological reactivity (orchids), as reflected by changes in blood pressure, heart rate, and cortisol levels, which make them highly sensitive to environmental change (Boyce & Ellis, 2005; Boyce, 2019).

A number of studies have examined the relation between biological reactivity and differential susceptibility to environmental influences (e.g., Ellis, Shirtcliff, et al., 2011; Manuck et al. 2011; Obradović et al., 2010), generally providing support for the orchid-dandelion distinction. For example, Obradović and her colleagues (2010) measured heart rate variability with respiration in 5- and 6-year-old children and related it to the quality of children's living conditions (e.g., income level, harshness of parenting, presence of maternal depression) and to their psychological adjustment. The authors reported that highly-reactive (orchid) children living in high-stress homes displayed poor psychological adjustment (for instance, poor school performance, increased externalizing behavior), whereas highly-reactive children from low-stress homes showed generally good adjustment. That is, orchid children flourished when early life conditions were positive but suffered when they were negative. In contrast, the less-sensitive dandelion children showed little difference in adjustment as a function of living conditions.

Other research has shown that children's temperament is a reasonable predictor of children's sensitivity to context, with orchid infants and children being more likely to have difficult temperaments and to be highly fearful and anxious than dandelion infants and children (e.g., Gilissen et al., 2008; Kochanska, 1993; Stright, Gallagher, & Kelly, 2008; see Belsky, 2005). A meta-analysis examining the findings of the relation between temperament, early living conditions, and psychological adjustment in 84 longitudinal studies supported the hypothesized relation between temperament and differential susceptibility: children with difficult temperaments (orchid children) living in supportive homes generally showed high levels of social and cognitive competence and low levels of internalizing and externalizing behaviors; in contrast, children with difficult temperaments living in high-stress homes, typified, for example by harsh parenting, showed, on average, much poorer adjustment (Slagt et al., 2016). Children with easy temperaments (dandelion children) were less affected by differences in quality of parenting. Other research has reported that children's sensitivity to context is associated with variants of specific genes (e.g., Bakermans-Kranenburg et al., 2008; Sumner et al., 2015), pointing to a clear genetic basis for at least some forms of differential susceptibility.

2.4 Domains of Mind

Earlier in this Element I referred to Geary's model of evolved psychological mechanisms (see Figure 1). To recapitulate, Geary proposed the mind is hierarchically organized, with two overarching domains, one dealing with social information (folk psychology) and the other dealing with ecological information. Each of these domains is composed of lower-level domains (the self, individual, and group for social; and biological and physical for ecological), which in turn consist of more specific domains (e.g., kin, in-group, out-group for the Group subdomain; movement, representation, tool-use for the Folk Physics domain). Infants enter the world not with fully formed cognitive mechanisms specific to a particular type of information, but rather with *skeletal competencies* that are fleshed out over development through exploration, play, and social interaction, that is through experience.

In the following sections I examine the development of some specific ecological and social skills and how an evolutionary perspective provides insight into their functioning. I first look at children's development of tool use. I spend most time on the development of a variety of social-cognitive abilities, primarily because I believe it was the evolution of social cognition that, more than other types of cognitive features, was responsible for the evolution of the modern human mind.

2.4.1 The Development of Folk Physics: Learning to Use Tools

When the topic of physics is mentioned, one might think of Isaac Newton or Albert Einstein. Rarely, do little children come to mind. Yet, early in life children need to deal with the basics of physics, including gravity, causality, and the various forms of matter. One reason for the long-time influence of Piaget's theory of intelligence is that he investigated infants' and young children's understanding of the physical world – the permanence of objects, the conservation of matter, and the understanding of space and time. What could be more essential for life than interacting with the physical world? There have been great debates about how these and other aspects of folk physics develop, and evolutionary developmental science has contributed to these discussions. For example, theorists taking an evolutionary perspective have proposed that infants come into the world with knowledge or processing constraints for particular domains, including the physical world and specifically representation of objects. This perspective, often referred to as *neonativism*, is reflected in concepts such as *core knowledge* (e.g., Spelke & Kinzler, 2007), *starting-state nativism* (Gopnik & Meltzoff, 1997), and the *principle of persistence* (Baillargeon, 2008). Consistent with Geary's concept of skeletal competencies, neonativists have shown that infants acquire a basic knowledge of the physical nature of objects gradually over infancy. Researchers have shown that young infants have a greater understanding of the constancy, cohesion, continuity, and permanence of objects than Piaget and others had proposed, and such understanding is based on impoverished knowledge of objects at birth that get fleshed out with experience over the first year of life (see Baillargeon, 2008; Baillargeon, Scott, & Bian, 2016; Spelke & Kinzler, 2007). Infants are not born as blank slates, but neither do they come into the world with a full-blown representation of objects. For that, experience is necessary.

One can argue that the development of object representation is important to varying degrees for most if not all vertebrates. However, one aspect of folk physics that is especially (if not uniquely) important to *Homo sapiens* is tool use. All human cultures involve the manufacture and use of artifacts, and many of those artifacts can be thought of as tools – artifacts created to solve specific problems. Humans are not the only tool-using species, but no other animal uses the variety of tools that humans do nor develops cultures so dependent on their use. Human children begin using tools early, and, just as children seem to have biases to develop an understanding of the cohesion and permanence of objects, they also seem to have inherited biases to learn to use tools.

Earlier in this section I noted that children learn about the affordances of objects and the rudiments of tool use through object-oriented play (e.g., Lockman, 2000; Smith, 1982), and that sex differences in object-oriented play may have been related to sex differences in tool use among our ancient ancestors (e.g., Geary, 2021). Tool use involves more than a familiarity with the physical properties of objects, however, but also with what a particular tool is *for*, and children from an early age seem to believe that every tool was designed for a specific purpose. Dennett (1990) referred to this as the *design stance*. For example, 12- and 18-month-old infants were shown a box with a hole on one side. The children then watched as an experimenter grasped the bulbous end of either a spoon or a novel object and inserted the slender end into the box, turning on a light. When infants were given an opportunity to turn the light on themselves, they successfully inserted the slender end of the novel object about 60 percent of the time, but were successful with the spoon only about 25 percent of the time, grasping instead the slender end and trying to insert the bulbous bowl-end into the hole. These infants had experience using spoons, and one holds a spoon by its slender end, hindering using the spoon in a novel way (Barrett, Davis, & Needham, 2007). In other research, 3-year-old children believe that an object designed for one purpose (e.g., catching bugs) is indeed a "bug catcher" even though it can be successfully used for another function (collecting raindrops) (Casler & Kelemen, 2005; see also Bloom & Markson, 1998; German & Johnson, 2002).

The design stance would seem to hinder children learning to use tools, as it results in a form of *functional fixedness*, the failure to identify alternative uses for familiar objects, which is also observed in adults (e.g., Duncker, 1945). Whereas the design stance may indeed hinder the flexible use of a tool, in more cases than not it would facilitate children learning a particular tool's function. Young children who observe or who are taught the use of a tool by a more competent member of their society can most readily learn its "proper" use by copying the model's actions in an appropriate context. Young children act as if they believe adults and older children know what a tool is for, which is likely true; the design stance affords children a short-cut way of mastering the most-likely function of that tool. According to Casler and Kelemen (2005, p. 479), "young children exhibit rapid learning for artifact function, already possessing an early foundation to some of our most remarkable capacities as tool manufac-turers and users." Although other species, including great apes, make and use tools, researchers have found no evidence that our simian relatives display the design stance (e.g., Buttelmann et al., 2008; Cummin-Sebree & Fragaszy, 2005; Ruiz & Santos, 2013).

It is interesting that young children's facility with learning to use tools does not seem to translate to tool innovation. A number of studies, including children from developed and traditional cultures (e.g., Bushman communities in south-ern Africa; Australian Aboriginal communities; Nielsen et al., 2014), have shown that preschool children perform especially poorly when they must modify simple tools (e.g., alter the shape of a flexible pipe cleaner to retrieve a desired object) to achieve a goal (e.g., Beck et al., 2011; Chappell et al., 2013). Cutting and her colleagues (2014) proposed that children may need more advanced cognitive abilities (e.g., memory, reasoning abilities) before they can create tools in contrast to their early-developing biases for learning to use tools. Stated another way, natural selection provided children with domain-specific adaptations for learning to use tools, but not for creating tools. Additional domain-general abilities are needed for tool innovation.

2.4.2 The Development of Folk Psychology and Hypersociality

Humans are a highly social species. In fact, *Homo sapiens* is a *hypersocial* species, akin to the eusocial insects – bees and ants. People have evolved the ability to function in large groups, cooperating with many different people – some of whom they may not know well or at all – to get difficult jobs done that an individual would not be able to accomplish alone. Humans evolved from social creatures, and our close genetic relatives, chimpanzees, are themselves highly social. Yet, human sociality substantially surpasses that of the great apes, and we see the beginnings of species differences in infancy and continuing into childhood (e.g., Rakoczy & Haun, 2020). In fact, Tomasello (2019, p. 6) asserted that "if we wish to explain how uniquely human psychology is created, we must focus our attention on ontogeny, and especially on how great ape ontogeny in general has been transformed into human ontogeny in particular."

In this section I examine some adaptations of infancy and childhood that are the basis for human hypersociality. To do this, I loosely follow Tomasello's (2019) *shared intentionality theory*. Tomasello proposed that two human-unique social-cognitive capacities emerge during infancy and childhood. The first, termed *joint intentionality*, develops in infancy and is first seen around nine months of age in *shared attention*. The second capacity is *collective intentionality*, in which children, beginning between 3- and 5-years of age, form a *group-minded "we"* with other people, resulting in the identification of in- and out-group members and social norms. In the following section I examine the development of several key social-cognitive adaptations of infancy and childhood, briefly noting how they differ from the abilities of great apes. These include shared attention and treating others as intentional agents; identifying and conforming to norms; prosociality; and collaboration.

Added to this list should be social learning. For example, although chimpanzees show a high degree of social learning, they rarely engage in *imitation*, understanding the goal of a model's actions and copying the actions of the model to achieve that goal. Rather, they are more likely to engage in *emulation*, in which they understand the goal of the model but use different behaviors to achieve that goal (e.g., Nagell, Olguin, & Tomasello, 1993; Horner & Whiten, 2005). In contrast, children, especially beginning around three years of age, are more apt to engage in true imitation, matching the model's behavior to achieve a similar goal. In particular, they engage in *overimitation*, duplicating as closely as possible all of a model's actions, even those that are seemingly unnecessary for task completion (e.g., Gellén & Buttelmann, 2019; see Hoehl et al., 2019; Whiten, 2019 for reviews). Overimitation, which persists into adulthood (e.g., McGuigan, Makinson, & Whiten, 2011), even in hunter-gatherer societies (e.g., Hewlett, Berl, & Roulette, 2016; Nielsen et al., 2016; Stengelin, Hepach, & Haun, 2020a, 2020b), fosters efficient acquisition of tool use for children (after all, the adults must know what they're doing), and reflects children's understanding and adoption of socially normative behaviors, including rituals. This is how "we" do it, and through overimitation children align themselves with their cultural group (e.g., Keupp, Behne, & Rakoczy, 2013; Legare & Nielsen, 2015; Nielsen, 2012). Such overimitation and increased attention to social others is not found in the great apes (e.g., Clay & Tennie, 2018; Nielsen, 2012) and sets the stage for a uniquely human form of social cognition.

Shared Attention and Treating Others as Intentional Agents

In shared attention, an infant and an adult partake in a triadic interaction with a third object or another person. For example, a father may point to and look toward an open door, and the infant will look in the direction of her father's gaze. They are sharing an experience (here, attention to an open door). It is the cognitive ability that underlies this seemingly simple interaction that transforms human social cognition. Infants are now treating people (here, a girl's father) as *intentional agents*, people who do things for a reason, or "on purpose." Infants understand that a referential gesture or gaze means that the gazer sees something that the infant does not, and that he or she wants the infant to see it as well. Dennett (1987) referred to this phenomenon as the *intentional stance*, in which people appeal to the mental states of others when attempting to explain what they do.

Shared attention increases into the second year, with infants now pointing to things that they want adults to pay attention to (e.g., Brooks & Meltzoff, 2002; Liszkowski, Carpenter, & Tomasello, 2007; Liszkowski et al., 2006). This developmental pattern is found in a wide range of cultures, including societies in which adults direct little attention to young infants (e.g., Callaghan et al., 2011), suggesting it is a species-typical adaptation that reliably emerges when infants experience a species-typical environment. Chimpanzees will sometimes follow the gaze of another ape, but there is no evidence that they engage in shared attention similar to that observed by 9-month-old human infants (e.g., Carpenter et al., 1995; Tomasello & Carpenter, 2005; Tomonaga et al., 2004). Treating others as intentional agents as reflected in shared attention may seem to be a relatively trivial cognitive accomplishment of infancy; but it is the basis of all more-advanced types of social cognition, including theory of mind, imitation, and teaching.

Identifying and Conforming to Social Norms

Conformity often gets a bad rap. How many parents have said to their child, in response to the statement, "But everybody else does it!", something to the effect, "If everybody jumped off a bridge, would you do it too?!" Yet a certain degree of conformity to group norms and behaviors is a good thing, a very good thing. Human cultures have much in common, but they also differ in important ways that define group membership, and fitting in with your group was a necessary survival skill for our ancestors and remains an important feature of human life today. Beginning around three years of age, children start to develop what Tomasello called *collective intentionality*, identifying not only with specific people with whom they have interacted, but with people, sometimes unknown to them, with whom they share some broader social commonality.

There is some hint of group-mindedness during the toddler years, with children selectively imitating same-sex as opposed to opposite-sex stereotypical behaviors (e.g., Bauer, 1993; Martin, Ruble, & Szkrybala, 2002); and 11- to 14-month-old children are more likely to imitate actions of a native speaker than a foreign speaker (e.g., Buttelmann et al., 2013; de Klerk et al., 2019) and to select food eaten by a native versus a foreign speaker (Shutts et al., 2009). True collective intentionality is seen when children begin to enforce group norms on others. This can be seen in the tattling of preschool children, who typically truthfully report rule violations of other children to teachers (Ingram, 2014; Ingram & Bering, 2010). Three-year-old children (but 5- and 6-year-old children more reliably) will give up some of their own resources (stickers, for example) to punish a cheater who violates the rules of a game (e.g., Riedl et al., 2015; Robbins & Rochat, 2011; Yang et al., 2018), but will punish out-group members more than in-group members (e.g., Jordan, McAuliffe, & Warneken, 2014). Even 9- to 14-month-old infants show a preference for interacting with individuals who treat others (especially in-group members) well as opposed to "wrong-doers" (e.g., Hamlin, Mahajan, Liberman, & Wynn, 2013; Tasimi & Wynne, 2016). Although chimpanzees and bonobos will retaliate against individuals that harm them, there is no evidence that they punish other apes for breaking social rules or for harming a third party (Reidl et al., 2012).

Young children seem to easily identify social groups (e.g., boys vs. girls; my family vs. your family; my classroom vs. your classroom) and often behave more favorably toward in-group members than toward out-group members. What is impressive is how little distinction is needed for children to identify in-groups from out-groups and to behave differentially. The *minimal groups paradigm*, originally developed with adults (Tafel et al., 1971), uses some arbitrary difference between two groups of people, such as the color t-shirts they wear, and examines how group membership affects children's behavior. In one study, 5-year-old children were assigned to wear either red or blue t-shirts and then shown photos of other children who were wearing either red or blue t-shirts. Children were asked how much they liked each pictured child, then told of either a positive or negative behavior and asked which child – the one wearing the red shirt or the one wearing the blue shirt – most likely committed the act. The children reported liking the in-group child (the one wearing the same color t-shirt as theirs) more than the out-group child; more frequently attributed positive behavior to the in-group child and negative behavior to the out-group child; and when given a chance to give coins to the two pictured children, gave more coins to the in-group than to the out-group child (Dunham, Baron, & Carey, 2011). This pattern of findings using the minimal groups paradigm has been replicated and extended many times, with preschool children showing more sharing, helping, trust in, and liking for in-group than for out-group members (e.g., Englemann et al., 2018; Patterson & Bigler, 2006; Plötner et al., 2015).

Tomasello described preschool children as *promiscuous normativists*. Young children in all cultures pay attention to social norms and group membership, although as they get older they vary how those rules are interpreted depending on the ecology and values of their culture (e.g., House et al., 2013). Children as young as three protest when arbitrary rules of a new game are violated and will point out when a puppet omits unnecessary actions on a tool-use task, protesting, for example, that the puppet is "doing it wrong" (e.g., Kenward, 2012; Keupp, Behne, & Rakoczy, 2013; Schmidt, Rakoczy, & Tomasello, 2016). Preschoolers are also more likely to imitate meaningless actions made by in-group than by out-group members (e.g., Gruber et al., 2019). Children's sensitivity to group norms and membership continues to develop into later childhood and adolescence and serves as the foundation for a unique form of sociality, qualitatively different than that seen in the great apes.

Prosociality

One important component of a hypersocial species is being nice to one another, and *Homo sapiens* is among the nicest of all primates. Cooperation demands that we sometimes put our immediate needs on hold so we can achieve a common goal, and this requires an unselfish, perhaps even altruistic, disposition. This is not to say that modern humans have given up their selfish ways. But our self-interested orientation is accompanied by prosocial actions, willing to help and share with others and to treat other people fairly. Such prosociality begins in early childhood and differentiates humans from the other great apes.

Consider helping. If you have spent much time with 3-year-olds, you know they always want to help – to crack an egg, to wash the dog, or hammer a nail (Rheingold, 1982). Most jobs would get done faster were the toddler not to help. In these circumstances, children's help may reflect a desire to be part of the group – to do what mom, dad, or a bigger sib is doing. Although adults in modern cultures often dissuade young children from helping too much, it is encouraged in most hunter-gatherer and traditional cultures, often leading into productive work. The effect is so robust that Lancy (2020) describes the time between about 14 months and 6 years as the "helper stage." By voluntarily and enthusiastically helping older people achieve some task, young children enhance their status in traditional societies toward full-fledged "personhood," develop important skills, and learn to share and cooperate with others.

Evidence from ethnographic research is supported by experimental work in modern cultures. For example, 14-month-old children watched with their parent as an unfamiliar adult tried to achieve some task, such as putting books into a closed cupboard or writing something with a marker. The children spontan-eously helped the adult without being asked, for example opening the cupboard door for the adult who had his hands full of books or retrieving a dropped marker. They did not offer help in similar situations when it seemed not to be warranted, for example the adult throwing the marker on the floor as opposed to accidently dropping it. Mother-raised chimpanzees put in similar situations did not offer help, although some enculturated chimps did (Warneken & Tomasello, 2006). The tendency for young children to help is quite robust, found across cultures (e.g., Corbit, Callaghan, & Svetlofa, 2020), with a number of studies reporting spontan-eous helping in toddlers and young preschoolers, with children being more likely to help familiar than unfamiliar people (e.g., Allen, Perry, & Kaufman, 2018; Hepach, 2016; Warneken & Tomasello, 2013; see Warneken, 2015 for a review).

Another prosocial behavior is sharing. Preschoolers are notoriously poor sharers, although in some conditions they are quite willing to share. For example, 18- and 24-month-old children were given four marbles to play a game. Children distributed the marbles evenly about half the time, and only monopolized all the marbles in 19 percent of the trials (Ulber, Hamann, & Tomasello, 2015). Children's sharing changes with age, with, for example, 3-year-olds being more likely than 2-year-olds to share with friends and with people who shared with them before (e.g., Olson & Spelke, 2008; Vaish, Hepach, & Tomasello, 2018), and children becoming more sensitive to social norms with age (e.g., sharing is what one is supposed to do in these situations; House & Tomasello, 2018). The tendency of preschoolers to share is similar across a wide range of cultures (e.g., Callaghan et al., 2011; Rochat et al., 2009; Samek et al., 2020), and both subsequent spontaneous helping and sharing are *negatively* associated with receiving rewards, suggesting that both are intrinsically motivated (e.g., Fabes et al., 1989; Ulber et al., 2016; Warneken & Tomasello, 2008).

Collaboration

It seems quite obvious that collaboration requires a prosocial disposition, but it also seems to require greater cognitive abilities than many preschoolers possess.

Just as there are predispositions toward conformity, helping, and sharing, are there similar early developing dispositions toward collaboration? The answer seems to be "yes." Under some circumstances, young children are able to work together to achieve a goal and then distribute the spoils of their efforts fairly.

Consider a study by Hamann and her colleagues (2011) in which 2- and 3-year-old children could get treats by pulling together ropes on either side of an apparatus. If only one child pulled, the treats remained out of reach; only by coordinating their actions would the treats be delivered, separately to each child. In some trials, the number of treats delivered differed between the children, with one lucky child getting three and the unlucky child getting only one. When this happened with 2-year-olds, the lucky children kept the three treats, leaving their cooperative partners with only a single treat. However, when 3-year-olds encountered the same situation, the lucky children shared the treats evenly with the unlucky children about 80 percent of the time. Such spontaneous sharing did not happen when treats were simply available to children when they entered the room, with one child having three treats and the other only one. It was only when these young children collaborated with one another to achieve a goal that they shared the treats fairly. When Hamann performed a similar experiment with adult chimpanzees, the apes rarely shared with their collaborative partner, acting like 2-year-old human children rather than the more fairness-minded 3-year-olds.

Although 2-year-olds may not equate collaboration with a sense of fairness, toddlers from diverse cultures will coordinate their behavior with an adult during a social game and will protest when an adult suddenly stops playing so the game can continue (Warneken, Chen, & Tomasello, 2006). Chimpanzees, in contrast, make no attempt to reengage an adult in a social game that has no food reward (Warneken et al., 2006). Other research testing 5- and 6-year-olds from Germany and Kenya reported that children from both countries were more likely to delay their gratification (eating a marshmallow) when completing a task that required cooperation with another child than when performing the task alone (Koomen, Grueneisen, & Herrmann, 2020), suggesting that children develop early the psychological disposition for collaboration.

Collaborating with another person requires that children treat their partners as intentional agents, take the perspective of their partner, and, according to Tomasello (2019), form a group-minded "we" with their partner. Children improve their collaborative skills with age, although even as toddlers they show early signs of cooperation. Children seemingly understand that collaborative effort deserves a fair distribution of rewards beginning around age three, with these skills continuing to improve throughout the preschool years. Although chimpanzees can also collaborate with one another to achieve a goal, they show no evidence of distributing the rewards of their efforts fairly, something that quickly results in a cessation of cooperation from the "unlucky" partner (e.g., Hamann et al. 2011).

The Developmental Origin of Hypersociality

Homo sapiens' hypersociality does not appear fully formed in adulthood but has its genesis in infancy and childhood. Young children have evolved biases to learn through observation, identify and follow social norms, behave prosocially toward others, and even to collaborate with conspecifics and treat their collaborative partners fairly. Although hints of hypersociality can be found in our close genetic relatives, chimpanzees, careful examination of these animals' social-cognitive skills reveals some significant differences. For example, researchers have examined differences between chimpanzees and human 2-year-olds on a wide range of problems, some involving tasks dealing with quantities, tools, and space (physical cognition) and others dealing with imitation, nonverbal communication, and reading the intentions of others (social cognition) (Hermann et al., 2007; Wobber et al., 2014). In these studies, chimps and children were comparable in most aspects of physical cognition, but children outperformed the apes on social cognition. Chimpanzees are smart animals, but their social cognition is qualitatively different from that of humans.

Human hypersociality emerged sometime over the past 5 to 7 million years, when humans last shared a common ancestor with chimpanzees. The origins of our species' unique sociality can be found early in development, based on modifications of great ape ontogeny. Children evolved social-cognitive adaptations that make learning the ways of one's social group almost inevitable, producing adults who can cooperate with one another to achieve tasks that are impossible to contemplate for any other species.

2.5 Developing Adaptations

Learning is essential for the success of long-lived, slow-developing animals, and this is especially true for *Homo sapiens*, and requires high levels of neural, cognitive, and behavioral plasticity. Plasticity is an evolved characteristic of humans, is "the rule" rather than the exception in evolution and development, and is greatest early in life. Infants and young children are sensitive to their circumstances, adjusting the trajectory of their development in anticipation of what their later environments might be like.

Natural selection has likely operated more potently at earlier than later stages of the lifespan, making infancy and early childhood the "crucible of natural selection." Humans, as all other species, have evolved adaptations to deal with recurrent problems faced by their ancestors, and these adaptations can be found across the lifespan. Some adaptations were necessary simply to keep the young organism alive at a particular time in development (adapting to the niche of childhood, ontogenetic adaptations), whereas others provided not only immediate but also deferred benefits (preparing children for adulthood, deferred adaptations).

Children are not born as blank slates, unconstrained by biology and able to adjust their behavior to whatever experiences they have. Rather, they seem to be *prepared* by natural selection to process some information more effectively than other information (e.g., language, tool use, some social relationships). However, one should not think of these adaptations as *innate* as the term is conventionally understood. Rather, *adaptations develop*, producing functional behaviors when a typically developing child experiences a species-typical environment. Different cultures use different tools, have different social norms, and different moral values. What does not differ among cultures is that children learn to use the technologies of their society, develop a sense of right and wrong, an understanding of the norms of one's social group, and, as Tomasello describes it, a group-minded "we." These early developing social abilities set the stage for an adult form of sociality and morality that has transformed the species and is in large part responsible for humans' domination of the planet.

3 How Can an Understanding of Human Development Help Us Better Understand Human Evolution?

Much like children today, our ancestors also developed, and changes occurring over the course of our forechildren's ontogeny served as the stuff on which natural selection worked. To quote biologist de Beer (1958, p. 1), "Embryos undergo development; ancestors have undergone evolution, but in their day they also were the products of development."

That our ancestors also developed may seem like an obvious truth, but for much of the twentieth century factors related to development were not seriously considered by mainstream evolutionary biologists. The primary reason for this was the realization that experiences of individuals during their lifetimes cannot become represented in the germ line (sperm and eggs) and thus could not be passed down to future generations. (No matter how many generations of mice have their tails cut off, tails persist.) Thus, from the perspective of evolution, development is an *epiphenomenon* – important to the individual and necessary to attain adulthood, but of no consequence to the evolution of the species. There were always a few scholars over the last century arguing that development did matter in evolution (e.g., Baldwin, 1902; de Beer, 1958; Garstang, 1922; Gottlieb, 1992; Gould, 1977), but theirs was a minority position. In the last few decades, the role of development in evolution has seen a revival, due to the emergence of the field of Evo Dev in biology (discussed later in this section) and developmental systems theory in developmental science (discussed in Section 2). In a significant way, and wholly within the Darwinian framework, development is taking a prominent role in evolutionary explication, including for *Homo sapiens*.

3.1 Developmental Plasticity as the Engine of Evolutionary Change and Epigenetic Theories of Evolution

In the previous section I emphasized the role of plasticity in human develop- ment and how infants' and children's abilities to modify their behavior in response to environmental context interact with evolved probabilistic cognitive mechanisms producing (usually) adaptive responses. The high degree of plasti- city shown by contemporary children was surely possessed by our forechildren, and changes in patterns of development in ancestral children, afforded by their high levels of plasticity, provided the variation on which natural selection operated. According to West-Eberhard (2003, p. 139): "Adaptive evolution [improvement in a species due to selection] is a two-step process: first the generation of variation by development, then the screening of that variation by selection."

For many biologists, the very idea that ontogeny plays an important role in phylogeny smacks of the discredited Lamarckian theory of the *inheritance of acquired characteristics*. Neither the necks of young giraffes nor the muscles of blacksmiths' children increase in size and strength due to the activities of their parents. Following the modern synthesis (the integration of Darwin's theory of evolution by natural selection with the genetic theory of inheritance), evolu- tionary changes were seen as the result of random mutations, which create the material on which natural selection operates. However, both earlier and more contemporary theory and research proposed alternative ways in which experi- ence during development can influence evolution while staying within the Darwinian tradition.

Perhaps the first such theory was that of developmental psychologist James Mark Baldwin (1896, 1902), who proposed that animals that had high levels of plasticity could modify their behavior in response to environmental stress resulting in enhanced survival relative to animals that enjoyed less develop- mental plasticity. This increased plasticity and responsivity could be passed along to offspring, giving future generations an adaptive advantage. Over many generations, these once-acquired behaviors become fixed and expressed without the need of a provoking environment, a process Baldwin called *organic selection*. Offspring do not so much inherit the acquired behavior of their parents, as in Lamarckism, but rather they inherit the genetic disposition to respond to stressful environments. Assuming the conditions that evoked the parents' adaptive responses continue to exist for the offspring, after repeated generations, the survival benefit of being able to adjust behavior to stressful environments (i.e., genetically based plasticity) will become fixed in the species, such that all members of the group express the adaptive behavior. From this perspective, genes (which Baldwin knew nothing about) still play a central role in evolutionary change, although it is behavior that takes the lead. Behavior is more susceptible to change (i.e., more plastic) than genes, especially early in life, and can respond quickly to environmental changes in disease, nutrition, predation, or climate (Mayr, 1982; Mayr & Provine, 1980).

Experimental support for Baldwin's theory (termed the *Baldwin effect*) came from studies by the mid-twentieth-century British biologist Waddington (1975). In a series of experiments, Waddington exposed fruit flies (*Drosophila melanogaster*) to heat shock or to a high-salt medium, which killed many animals but produced in survivors cross-veins in wings (in response to heat shock) or enlarged anal papillae (in response to being raised on a high-salt medium). The surviving flies were then crossbred with other survivors. After a number of generations, the new phenotypical characteristics (cross-veins or enlarged anal papillae) were expressed without the need of exposure to the initially provoking stimulus. Waddington (1975, p. 61) referred to this process of change as *genetic assimilation*, which he defined as "the conversion of an acquired character into an inherited one; or better, as a shift towards greater importance of heredity in the degree to which the character is acquired or inherited." Figure 3 provides a graphic sketch of the differences between Darwin's, Lamarck's, Baldwin's, and Waddington's theories of evolution. Natural selection plays the final role in determining evolutionary change in each theory except that of Lamarck.

Consistent with Waddington's findings, several researchers have proposed that changes in behavior as a result of response to novel environments are frequently the first step in evolutionary change, preceding genetic change (Gottlieb, 1987, 1992; West-Eberhard, 2003). For example, researchers in the 1960s reported transgenerational effects of experience in rats (Denenberg & Rosenberg, 1967; Ressler, 1966). Researchers cross-fostered some pups from two strains of rats (called C57BL and BALD), while other pups were raised by their own mothers (Ressler, 1966). When these animals were subsequently tested for learning ability, rats raised by BALD mothers – both those raised by their own BALD mothers and those C57BL rats cross-fostered by BALD mothers – displayed enhanced learning relative to rats

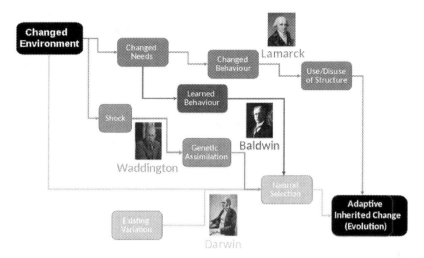

Figure 3 The Baldwin effect compared to Lamarck's theory of evolution, Darwinian evolution, and Waddington's genetic assimilation.
All the theories offer explanations of how organisms respond to a changed environment with adaptive inherited change. (Source : https://en.wikipedia.org/ wiki/File:Lamarck_Compared_to_Darwin,_Baldwin,_Waddington.svg. This file is licensed under the Creative Commons Attribution-Share Alike 4.0 International license.)

raised by C57BL mothers, and this effect persisted over two generations. There was something about how the BALD mothers raised their pups that affected their ability to learn. The researcher could not identify the mechanisms involved but suggested that "a nongenetic system of inheritance based upon transmission of parental influences is potentially available to all mammals" (Ressler, 1966, p. 267).

More recently, Meaney and his colleagues have shown that stress responses in rats can be transmitted across generations as a result of early rearing experiences. Rats that are frequently licked by their mothers display less stress as adults in an open-field setting than rat pups who are licked less often. When infant rats were cross-fostered – for instance, rats born to high-licking mothers but reared by low-licking mothers and vice versa – as adults they displayed the same pattern of response to stress and the same epigenetic markers as their *foster* mothers, not their *biological* mothers (e.g., Francis et al., 1999; Meaney, 2010, 2013). According to Meaney (2001, pp. 1170–1171), "Individual differences in behavioral and neuroendocrine responses to stress in rats are, in part, derived from naturally occurring variations in maternal care. Such effects might serve as a possible mechanism by which selected traits are transmitted from one generation to another."

Evidence for epigenetic inheritance in humans is less clear (but see Morgan & Whitelaw, 2008 for a discussion of possible epigenetic inheritance of diseases in humans). One well-documented but still controversial example of epigenetic inheritance in humans comes from a study that examined the effects of malnutrition on the children and grandchildren of women who were pregnant during the Dutch Hunger Winter of 1944–1945. Poor weather and Nazi policy during the waning years of World War II resulted in famine in the Netherlands. The children and grandchildren of women who were pregnant during the famine displayed life-long changes in methylation markers for genes linked with growth, development, and metabolism (Tobi et al., 2015). When the female offspring of the malnourished women became mothers themselves, their offspring had lower birthweights and ponderal indices (ratio of length to weight) than the offspring of adequately nourished mothers, and, later in life, were prone to obesity; they developed a metabolism that held onto calories, anticipating a postnatal environment similar in nutritional resources as their prenatal environment. That is, experiences of the grand-mother while pregnant influenced the development of her *grandchildren* (e.g., Lumey, 1992; Painter et al., 2008).

The theories of Baldwin, Waddington, and Meaney are examples of *epi-genetic theories of inheritance*, emphasizing the role of development in generating novel behaviors or responses to atypical or extreme environments. Such theories are not alternatives to Darwinian approaches but rather theories that recognize that changes during development produce the variation on which natural selection works. Animals have substantial genetic reserve that is only expressed under extreme or novel conditions, and, consistent with a conventional Darwinian approach, genes associated with survival and reproduction are passed on, resulting in increased survival of one's offspring. What differs from the perspective of the modern synthesis is the idea that environmentally provoked adaptabilities have a genetic basis, such that the experiences of an animal over its life course are also important to evolution. According to Konner (2010, p. 343), "At the leading edge of adaptation, experience during individual lives can establish a foothold for a new local dynamic of natural selection . . . Experience, far from being wasted because of the independence of the genome from the rest of the organism, pioneers what may become fundamental genetic changes." As noted in Section 2, the young of the species are most plastic, and this was surely true of our forechildren. As a result, it will often be children who discover new solutions to old problems or investigate, construct, and inhabit new niches, creating the stuff on which natural selection can work.

3.2 Maternal Effects

As noted repeatedly, plasticity – both for contemporary and ancestral popula-
tions – is greatest early in life. If you look back at the examples provided in this
and the previous sections, you will note that mothers are often the context for
such plasticity in young animals, whether it be for Gottlieb's ducks, the effects
of prenatal diet or stress, the rearing style of mother rats, or the lack of
"mothering" for institutionalized infants. For mammals in particular mothers
are *the* critical environment for infants, which also makes them the principal
environment of evolutionary change. Mothers serve as a buffer, or filter,
between infants and the external environment. Consistent with developmental
systems theory's idea of the bidirectionality of structure and function discussed
in Section 2, mothers not only contribute 50 percent of their offspring's genes,
but they influence their offspring's phenotypes through their behavior, which
influences genetic expression in the offspring, which in turn feeds back on the
infants, modifying infants' behavior and eventually the behavior of their
mothers (cf., Bornstein, 2009). This is graphically represented in Figure 4.

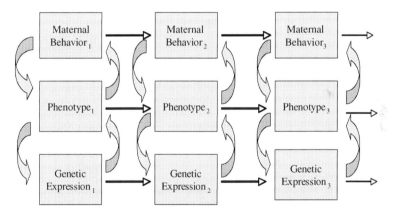

Figure 4 Maternal effects on offspring from a developmental systems
perspective (source: Bjorklund, 2006, with permission).

3.2.1 Obligatory Maternal Investment

It is trivial to say that "mothers matter." Research with a host of animals,
including humans, has unequivocally demonstrated the central role of mothers
on the outcomes of their children. For all mammals, this is due in part to the
obligatory investment that mothers make in their offspring in comparison to
that of fathers (Trivers, 1972). Conception and gestation occur within the
mother's body, and after birth it is only mothers who can provide nutrition in

the form of milk to the mammal infant. Following birth, mothers have the sole responsibility for rearing an infant to independence for 95 percent of mammal species, with humans being among the 5 percent of mammals in which males make some contribution to childcare. Although many modern fathers are devoting more time and effort to the care of their children than in generations past, mothers across the globe and throughout history (and surely prehistory) take responsibility for the bulk of childcare. According to Konner (2010), there is not a single traditional society in which fathers devote more time to childcare than mothers.

If it was change in the young that served as grist for the mill of natural selection, mothers were likely a critical part of the change-inducing environment. This means that differences in mothers may have induced changes in their highly plastic offspring, which is the first step in evolutionary change. From this perspective, plasticity to promote change is required not only for infants, but also for their mothers. For example, in the Netherlands, as a result of global warming, the caterpillars on which a species of bird (great tit, *Parus major*) feeds appear weeks earlier than in the past. As a result, most birds hatch too late to feed on the caterpillars, increasing the mortality rate of the young fledglings. Some females, however, had the plasticity to delay the timing of reproduction so their chicks hatched when the caterpillars were most plentiful and as a result those mothers had twice as many surviving offspring as birds not able to adjust their reproduction to the changing environment (Nussey et al., 2005).

3.2.2 Enculturated Apes

Perhaps more immediately relevant to human evolution is evidence that *Homo sapiens*' closest living relatives, chimpanzees (*Pan troglodytes*) and bonobos (*Pan paniscus*), alter some of their social-cognitive abilities to be more like that of human children when they are raised much as human children are reared. These *enculturated* apes are "mothered" by humans and experience early life much as human children would (Call & Tomasello, 1996). They are talked to, explicitly taught things (which mother apes rarely do), and engaged in *shared* (or *joint*) *attention*, as discussed earlier. The importance of such treatment is that enculturated apes are treated as *intentional agents* – as having wishes and desires that motivate their behavior and realizing that others' behavior is similarly motivated.

Social-cognitive abilities, as reflected by imitation, nonverbal communication, helping, and reading the intentions of others, are enhanced in enculturated great apes relative to mother- or laboratory-raised apes (e.g., Bjorklund et al.,

2002; Warneken & Tomasello, 2006). As I mentioned in the previous section, chimpanzees rarely engage in true imitation, copying the actions of the model to achieve that goal, but instead engage in *emulation*, in which they understand the goal of the model but use different behaviors to achieve that goal. The exception is for enculturated apes, which will imitate a human model's actions, both immediately and following a significant delay (Bering et al., 2000; Bjorklund et al., 2002; Buttelmann et al., 2007; Tomasello et al., 1993). In other words, when great apes experience a species-*atypical* early rearing environment, more like that of human children than that of mother-raised apes, they develop social-cognitive skills more similar to that of human preschoolers than that of apes. These young animals have the neural plasticity to alter important aspects of their social behavior as a result of modifications in "mothering." If ancestral apes had similar plasticity and latent social-cognitive abilities as displayed by modern apes, changes in parenting (with mothers surely doing most of it) could have prompted a change in the cognitive development of their offspring.

> If the environment responsible for the parenting change remained stable and if it affected multiple members of a population, it could have yielded a selective advantage for those individuals possessing enhanced social-learning skills. It would also have opened new niches for such individuals, perhaps promoting the transmission of social and technical (e.g., tool use) information and fostering new selective pressures that would further accelerate phylogenetic change (Bjorklund, 2006, p. 233).

Even if one believes that human technical skills were the leading edge for human evolution, such skills are most effectively acquired via social learning.

3.2.3 Social Complexity, Big Brains, and Slow Development

If ancient mothers played a role in modifying their offspring's behavior, cognition, and nervous system leading eventually to evolutionary change, it is highly likely that they did so in the realm of social cognition. Although there are many theories about how human intelligence evolved, one currently popular perspective is that social pressures were a driving engine for human cognitive evolution (e.g., Alexander, 1989; Dunbar, 2003; Whiten & Erdal, 2014). Most contemporary great apes are also social animals, as surely were our hominin ancestors. As I discussed earlier, humans, however, have evolved *hypersociality*, with the ability to interact and cooperate with conspecifics in both small and large groups. The *social brain hypothesis* contends that, as the social environments of our human ancestors became more complex, so did their need for social intelligence. Alexander (1989) went so far as to propose that humans invented their own selective pressure: themselves.

Child Development

But not just increased sociality led to the modern human mind; necessary accompaniments included a big brain and slow development. A large, slow developing brain afforded our ancestors the neural plasticity as well as the time to acquire the complex social skills that characterize all human groups (Bjorklund & Bering, 2003; Bjorklund, Cormier, & Rosenberg, 2005; Dunbar, 1995). Although humans are clearly the most socially and technologically complex species on the planet, other "intelligent" species, including elephants, cetaceans (dolphins and whales), and chimpanzees, also have relatively large brains, live in socially complex groups, and have a prolonged developmental period. The synergy among brain size, social complexity, and rate of development is illustrated in a study by Joffe (1997), who compared the size of the neocortex (the "thinking" part of the brain), social complexity (measured in terms of group size), and the length of the juvenile period for 27 different primate species, including human hunter-gatherers. Joffe reported strong correlations among these three factors: the bigger the brain relative to body size, the larger the social group, and the longer the juvenile period tended to be.

The proposal here is that ancestral mothers were the "environment" for their big-brained, slow developing, offspring, permitting them to acquire the social skills necessary to become effective members of their group. Once acquired, the enhanced sociality (particularly the ability to cooperate with group members) and social-learning skills could be applied to almost any problem – technical, social, or political – and mothers who promoted these abilities in their offspring would find their progeny at a decided advantage.

3.4 Evo Devo

The modern synthesis (or neoDarwinism) integrated Darwin's idea of natural selection with genetic theory. Evolution was the result of changes in gene frequencies, with natural selection favoring phenotypes with some combination of genes over other combinations. Genetic mutations were the proximal mechanisms by which new forms and functions were produced. In the twentieth century, evidence for evolution came primarily from the fields of genetics and paleontology. Gone was the idea favored by an earlier generation of biologists that changes in embryology had a significant role in evolution. What happened during the course of development was viewed as inconsequential to the evolution of the species. This view has changed with the advent of the field of *evolutionary developmental biology*, or *Evo Devo*. Evo Devo looks (mostly) at the embryonic development of different animals to infer their evolutionary relationship and how different developmental mechanisms affect species change (see Carroll, 2005; Raff, 1996).

At the core of Evo Devo is a set of four principles: modularity; the ancient origins of master genes; the role of regulatory genes in the evolution of body form; and heterochrony, genetic-based differences in developmental timing. *Modularity* refers to the fact that animals are composed of distinct units, or modules, with unique genetic specification, and natural selection can operate on different modules at different times. The circulatory system, for example, is distinct from the digestive system, and natural selection can operate independently on each system.

The second principle is the *ancient origins of master genes*. Genes that control sections of a body are similar in form across a wide range of animals, from fruit flies to humans. That is, these master genes, called *Hox* genes, control things such as the formation of eyes or appendages in a wide range of animals, although the type of eyes (compound eyes in insects, camera eyes in vertebrates) or appendages (legs, antennae, and wings in fruit flies; arms, legs, fingers, and vertebrae in animals with backbones) they produce depends on the species they are expressed in. Although it may seem strange that similar sets of genes are used to construct body parts in animals who last shared a common ancestor with one another 550 million years ago, the conservation of master genes may have been necessary for evolution to produce the diversity that it has. According to pioneering Evo Devo researcher Raff (1996, p. 27), "if each new species required the reinvention of control elements [master genes], there would not be time enough for much evolution at all, let alone spectacularly rapid evolution of novel features observed in the phylogenetic record. There is a kind of tinkering at work, in which the same regulatory elements are recombined into new developmental machines."

The third core principle of Evo Devo is *regulatory genes*, or genes that do not build bodies themselves, but turn on or turn off master (and other) genes. In fact, evolution may be due more to changes in regulatory genes than to protein-producing genes (see, e.g., Carroll, 2005; Noonan, 2003; Wray, 2007). For example, some of the largest genetic differences between chimpanzees and humans are found in regulatory genes associated with brain development (e.g., Arbiza et al., 2013; Gilad et al., 2006; McClean et al., 2011; Prabhakar et al., 2006).

One way in which regulatory genes can have a substantial impact in building bodies is by varying the time when master genes are activated. This brings us to the fourth core principle of Evo Devo, *heterochrony*, which refers to genetic-based differences in developmental timing. Recall the concept of modularity; different body parts are independent from one another, so that both regulatory genes and natural selection can operate on one module without affecting other modules. Genes associated with the development of a certain part of the body may be retarded or accelerated relative to the developmental rates experienced by a species' ancestors and can produce modifications in form or function that will then be subject to natural selection.[3]

One especially important type of heterochrony is *neoteny*, which refers to the slowing of development, or the retention of infantile or juvenile traits into later development. According to Montagu (1989, p. 246), "the evolutionary history of many groups, nonhuman and human, is characterized by delayed development, prolongation of the youthful stages into phases of sexual maturity, and the discarding of the old adult phase."

One impressive demonstration of neoteny at work comes from the research of Russian zoologist Dmitry Belyayev, who selectively bred wild red foxes (*Vulpes vulpes*) with the goal to make them dog-like pets, replicating the process that had converted wolves into domesticated dogs (see Trut, 1999; Trut, Oskina, & Kharlamova, 2009). Belyayev, and later his colleague Lyudmila Trut, selectively bred foxes that were initially friendly to humans, and after only 20 generations, 35 percent of foxes acted much like dogs, sniffing and licking humans and whimpering to gain attention, some as early as one month old. An unexpected side effect of selection for tameness was changes in body form. The domesticated foxes retained many of their puppy-like features into adulthood, including floppy ears, shortened legs, tails, snouts, and upper jaws, and shorter and wider heads. Trut and her colleagues (2009, p. 354) commented that, "The shifts in the timing of development brought about by selection of foxes for tameability have a neotenic-like tendency: the development of individual somatic [body] traits is decelerated, while sexual maturation is accelerated."

3.5 Humans as a Neotenous Species

Concerning human evolution, Carroll (2005, p. 267) wrote

> the picture of hominin evolution is a mosaic pattern, with different traits appearing at different times and evolving at different rates in hominin history ... the development of different structures was evolving in a patchy, nonlinear way over a long course of time. [O]ur history involved quantitative shifts in brain size, body proportions, skull size, gestation time, juvenile development, and more – assimilated over tens of thousands of generations.

---

[3] Technical note: Following McKinney and McNamara (1991), there are three types of heterochronic retardation: (1) *progenesis*, or earlier onset of some aspect of development; (2) *neoteny*, or reduced rate of development; and (3) *post-displacement*, or delayed onset of development. For ease of reading, I do not differentiate between these three types of retardation here, often using the term neoteny to refer to retardation of development in general. McKinney and McNamara also identified three forms of heterochronic acceleration: (1) *hypermorphosis*, or delayed offset of development; (2) *acceleration*, or increased rate of development; and (3) *pre-displacement*, or earlier onset of growth (from Bjorklund, 2007, p. 44).

Despite the fact that human evolution displays evidence of both acceleration and retardation of developmental rates relative to our ancestors for different systems, many scientists have proposed, dating back to the 1920s, that humans achieved many aspects of their form and function through the slowing of development, and view humans as a generally neotenous species (e.g., Bolk, 1926; Gould, 1977; Montagu, 1989). Humans' general neotenous nature is reflected by the Dutch Professor of human anatomy Louis Bolk (1926, p. 470), who wrote "There is no mammal that grows as slowly as man, and not one in which the full development is attained at such a long interval after birth . . . What is the essential in Man as an organism? The obvious answer is: The slow progress of his life's course."

Table 1 presents an abbreviated list of human neotenous traits. In the remainder of this section I will focus on two important neotenous features of *Homo sapiens* – brain development and the proposal that humans are a self-domesticated species, achieved through the retention of "tameness," much as displayed by Belyayev's foxes.

Table 1 Some neotenous functional traits in humans (adapted from Bjorklund, 2021, Bolk, 1926; Montagu, 1989; Skulachev et al., 2017)

Rapid growth of brain well into third year
Low birth weight
External gestation
Prolonged immaturity
Prolonged dependency
Infant's great need of fluids (150 ml per day)
Fetal rate of bodily growth, weight, and length during first year
Prolonged growth period
Ends of long and finger/toe bones remain cartilaginous for years
Late development of reproductive maturity
Small nose
Longer legs than arms
Absence of baculum (penis bone)
How the spine connects to the base of the skull, permitting bipedal locomotion
Orientation of the vagina

3.5.1 Brain Development

Perhaps the most significant physical difference between modern humans and our closest relative, chimpanzees, is the size of our brains relative to body size. This difference in brain size is also surely related to the substantial social and cognitive differences between the species as well. Clearly, *Homo sapiens'* brains evolved to be larger than those of our ancient ancestors, but they did so by retaining the rapid prenatal rate of development typical of primates into postnatal life. As noted previously, there was selective pressure on ancient hominins to build larger brains, possibly to deal with the increasing complexity of social life. However, the fetal brain could get only so large before it could not fit through the birth canal of a bipedal woman. (Upright stance evolved before brain expansion in hominins.) The solution to this conundrum, the so-called *obstetrical dilemma* (Washburn, 1960), was for children to be born early, relative to the typical primate schedule, with brain development that would normally occur before birth in a comparably sized primate occurring after birth in our human ancestors. At birth, human brains are about 28 percent of their eventual adult weight. In comparison, the brains of contemporary great apes are between about 40 percent and 45 percent of their eventual adult weight (DeSilva, 2016; Trevathan & Rosenberg, 2016), meaning that more brain development (in terms of neuron size and formation of synapses) occurs after birth for humans than for the other apes. If human infants followed the typical primate schedule of brain development, gestation could last 18 to 24 months.

As a result of retaining the prenatal rate of growth into the second year of life, human infants' brains develop in a physically, perceptually, cognitively, and socially richer environment than do the brains of other great apes. They are exposed to a world of sights, sounds, and people, and these experiences surely influence subsequent brain development (see Portmann, 1990; Montagu, 1989; Konner, 2010). Portmann (1990) argued that this period of rapid postnatal brain development, which he called the *extrauterine spring*, contributed to the unique set of social and cognitive abilities characteristic of *Homo sapiens*. Imagine, Portmann (1990) asked, "the developing human spending the important maturation period of its first year in the dark, moist, uniform warmth of its mother's womb . . . It will gradually become clear that world-open behavior of the mature form is directly related to early contact with the richness of the world, an opportunity available only to humans" (p. 93).

There is also evidence of neoteny affecting the development of individual neurons in the human brain, especially with respect to neuronal plasticity. Neuronal metabolism and synaptic activity peak later in humans than in other primates (see, e.g., Bufill et al., 2011; Charrier et al., 2012; Liu et al., 2012; Petanjek et al., 2011), as does the process of myelination (Miller et al., 2012), thus extending neural plasticity into adulthood. In their review of neuronal neoteny, neuroscientists Bufill, Agustí, and Blesa (2011, p. 735) wrote,

> human neurons belonging to particular association areas retain juvenile characteristic throughout adulthood, which suggests that a neuronal neoteny has occurred in *H. sapiens*, which allows the human brain to function, to

a certain degree, like a juvenile brain during adult life . . . Neuronal neoteny contributes to increasing information storage and processing capacity throughout life, which is why it was selected during primate evolution and, to a much greater extent, during the evolution of the genus *Homo*.

3.5.2 Humans as a Self-Domesticated Species

When we speak of domesticating animals, we typically mean making wild animals tame. Recall that when Belyayev selectively bred wild foxes for tameness, neotenous physical features came along with the behavioral changes. A number of theorists have proposed that *Homo sapiens* is a *self-domesticated species*, in which neotenous behaviors were selected for increased prosociality and cooperativeness (or "survival of the friendliest" to use Hare's phrase; see, e.g., Bjorklund, 2021, in press; Hare, 2017; Hood, 2014; Wrangham, 2019). Specifically, humans retain the juvenile feature of reduced levels of *reactive aggression*, which occurs in response to real or perceived threat. Although no one should view *Homo sapiens* as a peaceful species, compared to chimpanzees and other social apes, humans display relatively low levels of reactive aggression, although they display high levels of premeditated *proactive*, or instrumental, *aggression*. Reduced levels of reactive aggression are associated with increased inhibition, the ability *not* to respond to an immediate stimulus, with several theorists proposing that humans' enhanced sociality was mediated by an increase in inhibition (see, e.g., Bjorklund & Harnishfeger, 1995; Chance, 1962; Stenhouse, 1974).

Although reduced reactive aggression and enhanced inhibition abilities likely provided a number of advantages for our ancestors (e.g., greater control of male sexual urges; ability to deceive others to gain social advantages; increased ability to delay gratification), perhaps the greatest advantage was associated with the ability to cooperate with fellow group members to achieve a common goal. As mentioned previously, hypersociality is a hallmark of our species, and hypersociality can only evolve in an animal capable of working peacefully with conspecifics long enough to get a job done. This does not mean that humans must forego the benefits of aggression in achieving their goals. In fact, Wrangham (2019) proposed that ancient humans used proactive aggression to control (and sometimes kill) bullies and other individuals who violated group norms.

3.6 New Stages of Development

Humans take a long time to reach sexual maturity, longer than any other mammal. Animals that take a long time to reach adulthood also tend to live longer, but humans' extended period of immaturity is exaggerated relative to other long-lived and slow-developing animals, such as elephants, dolphins, and chimpanzees. There is great cost to waiting so long to reproduce, chiefly the possibility of dying. In biology, when there is great cost to an adaptation there must be great benefit, otherwise natural selection would have eliminated the feature. One proposal for the adaptive value of *Homo sapiens*' slow development is the need to learn the complexities of human social groups. However, our ancestors not only prolonged their pre-reproductive period, but, according to Bogin (1999, 2003), developed new stages of development in the process, in large part to deal with the increasing complexity of the social environment.

All mammals go through at least three stages of development: infancy, extending from birth to weaning; the juvenile period, extending from the onset of weaning to sexual maturity; and adulthood. Mammal infants are highly dependent on their parents (mostly their mothers) for food and protection. Juveniles become increasingly independent from their mothers, typically fend for themselves in terms of nutrition, and, in social species, play or otherwise interact with fellow juveniles. Humans also go through these three stages, but Bogin claims *Homo sapiens* evolved two additional stages on their way to adulthood: childhood and adolescence.

In traditional cultures, human infants are typically breastfed until about three years of age. According to Bogin, weaning is followed by the new stage of *childhood*, extending from about 3 to about 7 years. During childhood, children in hunter-gatherer cultures have greater independence from their parents, spend much of their time in mixed-age play groups, but are still dependent on adults for food (they have baby teeth and lack the skills to forage or hunt), and, although displaying substantially greater intelligence than infants, still show a form of cognitive immaturity, captured by Piaget's description of children during the preoperational stage of development.

Children during the *juvenile period* (often referred to as middle childhood by psychologists and educators) have greater independence, more advanced forms of thinking, and although they remain dependent on adults for survival in all cultures, they are able to take care of themselves far better than preschool-age children. Many juveniles in modern societies get themselves to and from school with little help, prepare simple meals at home, and generally have increasing strength, dexterity, and cognitive abilities approximately those of adults. In fact, many juveniles manage to eke out an existence in groups of other children as "street kids" in cities and villages on every continent of the world.

The new stage of *adolescence* begins with the growth spurt shown by both girls and boys and is characterized by a period of low fertility for females. Research has also demonstrated changes in brain organization during

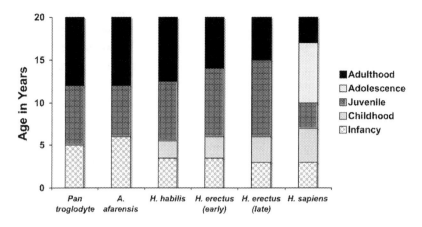

Figure 5 Evolution of human life-history stages. According to Bogin, humans
evolved two new life stages: childhood and adolescence
(source: Bogin, 2001, reprinted with permission).

adolescence, with the amount of gray matter decreasing (reflective of the
pruning of neuronal cell bodies), the amount of white matter increasing (reflective of myelination of axons in the frontal cortex), and the distribution of
neurotransmitters, such as dopamine and serotonin, changing between the
juvenile and adolescent stages in both the limbic system and the frontal cortex
(see Dennis et al., 2013; Giedd, 2015; Giedd et al., 1999; Spear, 2007). In
addition, many structures in the limbic system (associated with emotion) reach
adult levels of functioning before the prefrontal lobes (the area involved in
higher-order cognition as well as inhibition and self-regulation of behavior),
causing what some researchers refer to as a mismatch in maturation (Giedd,
2015; Mills et al., 2014). Although subadult animals of other species are
sometimes referred to as "adolescents," no other species displays the rapid
growth spurt and brain reorganization typical of humans.

Based on fossil evidence, Bogin suggested that the stages of childhood and
adolescence evolved gradually over hominin evolution. Figure 5 presents the
proposed life stages for modern chimpanzees (*Pan troglodytes*), *Australopithecus
afarensis*, *Homo habilis*, early and late *Homo erectus*, and *Homo sapiens*.[4] Bogin

---

[4] Humans last shared a common ancestor with contemporary chimpanzees and bonobos between 5
and 7 million years ago. Over that time, there existed in Africa a series of *hominin* species, a group
consisting of modern humans, extinct human species, and all of humans' immediate forebearers.
Australopithecus afarensis lived in Africa, walked upright much as humans do, but had a skull the
size of a chimpanzee. *Homo habilis* (Handy Man), the first member of the *Homo* genus, lived in
eastern Africa, had a larger brain, and developed a stone-tool technology referred to as Olduwan.
Homo erectus (or *Homo ergaster*) had a larger brain still, developed a more sophisticated stone
tool kit called Acheulean, and about 1.8 million years ago some members of the species left Africa

proposed that the first evidence of childhood can be found in *Homo habilis*, about 2.5 million years ago, with the length of childhood increasing in *Homo erectus* and *Homo sapiens*. Bogin identified the first signs of adolescence in *Homo sapiens*.

Bogin proposed that these new stages, with their associated social and cognitive characteristics, must have provided some adaptive advantages to ancient children. With respect to childhood, although 3- to 7-year-old children are no mental giants, they possess the beginnings of a cognition that is qualitatively (or at least massively quantitatively) different from that of any other animal. They become symbol users, using language to communicate not only about the present but also to talk about the past and the future. Early in childhood, children engage in *counterfactual thinking* – creating something that is "counter to the facts." As discussed in an earlier section, this is the basis of sociodramatic play, apparent in most 3-year-olds, in which children take on different roles and follow a story line as if they were in a theatrical performance. Nielsen (2012) proposed that counterfactual thinking is a central feature of human childhood that played a critical role in the evolution of human cognition, and that "by pretending children thus develop a capacity to generate and reason with novel suppositions and imaginary scenarios, and in so doing may get to practice the creative process that underpins innovation in adulthood" (p. 176). Also developing during this time are children's increasing social-learning abilities, discussed earlier. According to Nielsen (2018, p. 266), "Children show they are prepared socially and cognitively to adopt the ritualized behaviors of those around them in many ways … the most compelling of which is overimitation."

Human adolescence is associated with advances in cognition, but also with an increasing quest for independence and agency. This quest for independence is often reflected in increased risk-taking and novelty seeking and greater self- and social awareness. Few, if any, cultures treat adolescents as true adults (despite some ceremonies to the contrary), and the changes associated with adolescence likely foster further separation of youth from their parents and help establish their place in their social group in a relatively low-risk environment.

3.7 Ontogeny and Phylogeny

Humans evolved from big-brained, slow-developing, social animals, with each of these characteristics reaching its zenith in *Homo sapiens*. The young of

---

and populated much of Europe and Asia. Modern *Homo sapiens* evolved in Africa as early as 300,000 years ago, with some migrating into Europe and Asia between 50,000 and 100,000 years ago, where they outcompeted or exterminated other *Homo* species (*Homo erectus*, *Homo neanderthalensis*) they encountered.

ancient humans and of our hominin ancestors displayed substantial levels of neural, cognitive, and behavioral plasticity, and changes in early development in response to early environments led the way to evolutionary change. There is no need for a hocus-pocus Lamarckian explanation for this process: Animals that had the genes associated with high levels of plasticity were more apt to survive than animals with less-plastic genomes, passing these qualities on to their offspring. Many of these changes likely occurred in the presence of an animal's mother, both pre- and postnatally, with mothers essentially being the effective environment for young mammals.

Genetic-based changes in rates of early development also had a strong effect on the evolution of *Homo sapiens*, with neoteny having a particularly profound influence. Ancient hominins' reductions in reactive aggression possibly permitted the evolution of hypersociality, and the retention of prenatal brain growth rates into postnatal life transformed human sociality and cognition. The necessity of human infants' "early" birth results in our experiencing a vastly more complex physical, perceptual, social, and cognitive world than would be the case if we followed the typical ape trajectory of brain development. From this perspective, the mammalian stage of infancy is different in humans from that of other primates. And while infancy may not be a new mammalian stage, that of childhood and adolescence seemingly were, and each was necessary for the substantial social-cognitive changes that occurred in hominin evolution to produce the culturally and technologically unique species we have become.

4 Children, Childhood, and Development in Evolutionary Perspective

Children have been developing since time immemorial, and how they developed determined the adults they grew into. The process of development has not been static, however, but has changed over evolutionary time, with infants and children being shaped by natural selection to produce the species we are today.

For most of the history of developmental science, Darwinian theory has been an outsider to explaining or understanding psychological development. This has changed in recent decades, with many psychologists recognizing that an evolutionary developmental perspective can provide great insights into children, childhood, and the adults children become.

4.1 The Biologizing of Development

The advent of evolutionary developmental science was part of an increasing biologizing of development extending back at least to the 1990s. It perhaps should not be surprising that developmental scientists were quick to recognize and focus on the importance of biological factors, in that *development* itself is a biological concept. Development is characteristic of the species, has its basis in biology, and is relatively predictable, at least broadly speaking. Yet, there is enough variability on the path to adulthood that any child takes to make it interesting, and understanding the underlying biology of these changes can be greatly informing. As such, developmental scientists quickly accepted research into the underlying biological proximal causes of development and its variation, especially developmental neuroscience (e.g., Byrne & Fox, 1998; Marshall, 2015). Research demonstrating how experience affects brain and psychological development were easily incorporated into the mainstream paradigms of developmental science. Research into behavioral epigenetics has recently attracted the attention of developmental scientists, providing biological explanations for how experience alters gene expression and thus behavior (e.g., Conradt, 2017; Moore, 2015).

Developmentalists were less enthusiastic about biologically distal explanations of development, however, as exemplified by evolutionary theory. In an essay written as part of the 100th anniversary of the founding of the American Psychological Association, Charlesworth (1992) stated that Darwin had had little influence on developmental psychology. Although early developmental scientists including Piaget, Pryor, Freud, and Werner had incorporated evolutionary concepts into their theories, many of these concepts were preDarwinian, often emphasizing discredited ideas such as the recapitulation theory of the nineteenth-century biologist Ernst Haeckel ("ontogeny recapitulates phylogeny"; see also Morss, 1990). Charlesworth attributed Darwin's minimal influence as due to the theory's perceived incompatibility with developmentalists' emphasis on *meliorism*, the fostering of development. Evolutionary theory was seen as endorsing a form of *genetic determinism*, with the implication of the immutability of behavior, the antithesis of meliorism. As I hope has been clear in the pages of this Element, evolutionary developmental psychology does not advocate such a static perspective and instead emphasizes that dynamic developmental plasticity is an evolved feature of *Homo sapiens*.

Over the past three decades evolutionary accounts of development have been increasingly accepted by mainstream scientists (although not by all; see, e.g., Witherington & Lickliter, 2016). Infants and children have been prepared by natural selection for life in a human group. They are not born as blank slates but possess skeletal psychological mechanisms related to physical and social domains, such that infants process some information more readily than others. These mechanisms should not be viewed as "instincts" or as being "innate," in that they require experience for their proper expression. Prepared is not preformed. Some of these mechanisms evolved to adapt children to their immediate environment and disappear or are modified once no longer needed (ontogenetic adaptations), whereas others serve to prepare children for life as adults (deferred adaptations). Such adaptations can account for universal aspects of development as well as individual differences observed among children, both within and across cultures.

4.2 Self-Socialization of Human Development and Evolution

As suggested in this Element, infants and children come equipped with evolved probabilistic cognitive mechanisms, arising from low-level cognitive and perceptual abilities. Such mechanisms develop into adaptive behavior and thought when children experience a species-typical environment. The probabilistic nature of these mechanisms implies a high degree of plasticity, which is necessary for children to adjust their behavior to a particular social setting, or for the development of atypical and possibly pathological behavior (and its modification) should children experience a species-atypical environment.

The nature of evolved probabilistic cognitive mechanisms also means that children will acquire important skills, values, and norms of their culture without the need of specific tutorials. In most Western cultures we talk of "teaching" children even for the most basic cognitive skills and social norms. In contrast, adults in traditional cultures do little direct teaching, yet children acquire the ways of their society as readily as do children for whom direct instruction is the norm. Children's evolved and inherited adaptations cause them to be especially attentive to important aspects of their physical and social environments and to adopt those behaviors and norms without the need of direct instruction. Children learn to use a culture's tools by observation and by acting as though more experienced people know what they are doing when using a tool. Once exposed to a tool, children assume it is used for a specific purpose (the design stance) and will copy both the necessary and unnecessary actions of a model when using a tool or engaging in some ritual (overimitation). Children's strong tendency to look for and adopt conventional cultural norms (promiscuous normativity) results in their identification of in-groups and out-groups and adopting the behaviors and values of the in-group. The lack of need of direct instruction in acquiring social norms can be seen in children's acquisition of gender roles in all cultures (even those cultures that attempt to minimize such roles) as well as the ease with which children reward, punish, imitate, and evaluate in- versus out-group members, often based on minimal features (such as the color t-shirt one is assigned). In essence, children's evolved probabilistic cognitive mechanisms result in their *self-socialization* to their particular culture.

Such self-socialization also surely characterized our forechildren and may have had important consequences for human evolution. Some theorists proposed that *Homo sapiens* is a self-domesticated species. Much as humans domesticated livestock and dogs, producing tamer and more neotenous animals, so too did ancient humans alter their own development, retaining juvenile aspects of behavior and becoming more prosocial and cooperative. Through neoteny, humans reduced their levels of reactive aggression and as a result produced a species that could increasingly cooperate with conspecifics to achieve a common goal and the eventual evolution of hypersociality. Although it is typically adults who collaborate with one another to achieve goals unattainable by any single person, it was surely the self-socializing abilities of ancient children that set the stage for adult hypersociality.

4.3 Conclusions

There can be little doubt that *Homo sapiens'* unique social, emotional, and cognitive abilities are the products of evolution by natural selection. Perhaps we should not make too much of this obvious truth, for each extant species is unique and the product of its natural selection. Yet, we have a self-interest in understanding the origins of our own species, and our species is special to the extent that, for better or worse, we hold hegemony over the planet on which we reside.

An evolutionary perspective of development represents not only a particular account of ontogeny, but a *metatheory* for development, a broader framework for more specific theories that organizes known facts parsimoniously, provides guidance to important domains, and unifies the study of development with the rest of the life sciences. An evolutionary perspective goes beyond describing ontogeny, asking why we develop the way we do, leading to investigating the processes that govern development. As social psychologist Kurt Lewin (1943) noted, there is nothing as practical as a good theory, and this may be especially true of a good metatheory.

In addition to enhancing developmental science, an evolutionary perspective on development can help explain, and occasionally solve, some of the problems of modern life faced by our children. This may be best reflected by the *mismatch hypothesis*, the idea that there is a mismatch between children's evolved adaptations, formed in ancient environments, and their current circumstances (Bjorklund, 2021). Some of these mismatches can be found in the practices of well-intentioned parents from WEIRD cultures, being overprotective of their children (practicing "safetyism," Lukianoff & Haidt, 2018). Such overprotection can result in their children following an exaggeratedly slow life history strategy, resulting in young people being less prepared for adult life than previous generations. Other mismatches are related to modern technology and the need for formal schooling. Social media can be viewed as a superstimulus, providing both matches and mismatches with adolescents' and young adults' evolved drives for social interaction and belonging, affording both opportunities to enrich life and to conditions producing increased levels of depression and anxiety (Bjorklund, 2021). Formal schooling represents a mismatch with how our forechildren learned. Evolutionary theory can suggest better ways to educate children by providing materials and situations that match children's evolved biases to make sense of information, and by structuring schools to better match children's and adolescents' evolved adaptations for learning (e.g., Geary & Berch, 2016; Gray, 2016; Wilson, Kauffman, & Purdy, 2011). Solutions to bullying in school are more likely to be achieved when programs recognize the adaptive benefits of bullying for the bully in terms of reputation and status, particularly for the social-conscious adolescent (e.g., Ellis et al., 2016; Yeager, Dahl, & Dweck, 2018). An evolutionary perspective may not be necessary for dealing with problems modern children face, but by identifying these mismatches parents, educators, and policy makers can better improve the lives of children and the adults they will become.

The primary message in this Element is that it is not sufficient to take only an evolutionary or only a developmental perspective to attain a better understanding of human childhood, but that the two must be combined. Infants and children have been the target of natural selection as much as or more so than adults. Just as an evolutionary perspective can give us greater insights into child development, so also can an evolutionary developmental perspective provide greater insight into both the adults we become and the species we became.

References

Alexander, R. D. (1989). Evolution of the human psyche. In P. Mellers and C. Stringer (Eds.), *The Human Revolution: Behavioural and Biological Perspectives on the Origins of Modern Humans.* Princeton, NJ: Princeton University Press, pp. 455–513.

Allen, M., Perry, C., & Kaufman, J. (2018). Toddlers prefer to help familiar people. *Journal of Experimental Child Psychology, 174*, 90–102. https://doi .org/10.1016/j.jecp.2018.05.009

Anzures, G., Wheeler, A., Quinn, P. C., Pascalis, O., Slater, A. M., Heron-Delaney, M., Tanaka, J. W., & Lee, K. (2012). Brief daily exposure to Asian females reverses perceptual narrowing for Asian faces in Caucasian infants. *Journal of Experimental Child Psychology, 112*, 484–495. https://doi.org/10 .1016/j.jecp.2012.04.005

Arbiza, L., Gronau, I., Aksoy, B. A., Hubisz, M. J., Gulko, B., Keinan, A., & Siepel, A. (2013). Genome-wide inference of natural selection on human transcription factor binding sites. *Nature Genetics, 45*, 723–729. https://doi .org/10.1038/ng.2658

Baillargeon, R. (2008). Innate ideas revisited: For a principle of persistence in infants' physical reasoning. *Perspectives on Psychological Science, 3*, 2–13. https://doi.org/10.1111/j.1745–6916.2008.00056.x

Baillargeon, R., Scott, R., & Bian, L. (2016). Psychological reasoning in infancy. *Annual Review of Psychology, 67*, 159–186. https://doi.org/10 .1146/annurev-psych-010213–115033

Bakermans-Kranenburg, M. J., van IJzendoorn, M. H., Pijlman, F. T., Mesman, J., & Juffer, F. (2008). Experimental evidence for differential susceptibility: Dopamine D4 receptor polymorphism (DRD4 VNTR) moderates intervention effects on toddlers' externalizing behavior in a randomized controlled trial. *Developmental Psychology, 44*, 293–300. https://doi.org/10 .1037/0012–1649.44.1.293

Baldwin, J. M. (1896). A new factor in evolution. *American Naturalist, 30*, 441–451; 536–553. https://doi.org/10.1086/276408

Baldwin, J. M. (1902). *Development and Evolution.* New York, NY: McMillan.

Bandura, A. (1997). *Self-efficacy: The Exercise of Control.* New York, NY: Freeman.

Barker, J. E., Semenov, A. D., Michaelson, L., Provan, L. S., Snyder, H. R., & Munakata, Y. (2014). Less-structured time in children's daily lives predicts self-directed executive functioning. *Frontiers in Psychology, 5*, 1–16. https:// doi.org/10.3389/fpsyg.2014.00593

Barrett, T. M., Davis, E. F., & Needham, A. (2007). Learning about tools in infancy. *Developmental Psychology, 43*, 352–368. https://doi.org/10.1037 /0012–1649.43.2.352

Bateson, P. (2002). The corpse of a wearisome debate. *Science, 297*, 2212–2213. https://doi.org/10.1126/science.1075989

Bauer, P. J. (1993). Memory for gender-consistent and gender-inconsistent event sequences by twenty-five-month-old children. *Child Development, 64*, 285–297. https://doi.org/10.2307/1131452

Beck, S. R., Apperly, I. A., Chappell, C., Guthrie, C., & Cutting, N. (2011). Making tools isn't child's play. *Cognition, 119*, 301–306. https://doi.org/10 .1016/j.cognition.2011.01.003

Beckett, C., Maughan, B., Rutter, M., Castle, J., Colvert, E., Groothues, C., Kreppner, J., Stevens, S., O'Connor, T. G., & Sonuga-Barke, E. J. S. (2006). Do the effects of early severe deprivation on cognition persist into early adolescence? Findings from the English and Romanian Adoptee Study. *Child Development, 77*, 696–711. https://doi.org/10.1111/j.1467–8624 .2006.00898.x

Belsky, J. (2005). Differential susceptibility to rearing influence. In B. J. Ellis and D. F. Bjorklund (Eds.), *Origins of the Social Mind: Evolutionary Psychology and Child Development*. New York, NY: Guilford, pp. 139–163.

Belsky, J. (2019). Early-life adversity accelerates child and adolescent development. *Current Directions in Psychological Science, 28*, 241–246. https://doi.org/10.1177/0963721419837670

Belsky, J., & Pluess, M. (2009) Beyond diathesis–stress: Differential suscepti-bility to environmental influence.*Psychological Bulletin, 135*, 885–908. https://doi.org/10.1037/a0017376

Belsky, J., Steinberg, L., & Draper, P. (1991). Childhood experience, interper-sonal development, and reproductive strategy: An evolutionary theory of socialization. *Child Development, 62*, 647–670. https://doi.org/10.2307 /1131166

Bering, J. M., Bjorklund, D. F., & Ragan, P. (2000). Deferred imitation of object-related actions in human-reared juvenile chimpanzees and orangutans. *Developmental Psychobiology, 36*, 218–232. https://doi.org/10 .1002/(SICI)1098–2302

Bick, J., Zeanah, C. H., Fox, N. A., & Nelson, C. A. (2018). Memory and executive functioning in 12-year-old children with a history of institutional rearing. *Child Development, 89*, 495–508. https://doi.org/10.1111/cdev .12952

Bjorklund, D. F. (1987). A note on neonatal imitation. *Developmental Review, 7*, 86–92. https://doi.org/10.1016/0273–2297(87)90006–2

Bjorklund, D. F. (1997). The role of immaturity in human development. *Psychological Bulletin, 122*, 153–169. https://doi.org/10.1037/0033-2909 .122.2.153

Bjorklund, D. F. (2003). Evolutionary psychology from a developmental systems perspective: Comment on Lickliter and Honeycutt (2003). *Psychological Bulletin, 129*, 836–841. https//doi:10.1037/0033-2909.129.6.836

Bjorklund, D. F. (2006). Mother knows best: Epigenetic inheritance, maternal effects, and the evolution of human intelligence. *Developmental Review, 26*, 213–42. https://doi.org/10.1016/j.dr.2006.02.007

Bjorklund, D. F. (2007). *Why Youth is* Not *Wasted on the Young: Immaturity in Human Development*. Oxford: Blackwell.

Bjorklund, D. F. (2015). Developing adaptations. *Developmental Review, 38*, 13–35. https://doi.org/10.1016/j.dr.2015.07.002

Bjorklund, D. F. (2016). Prepared is not preformed: Comment on Witherington and Lickliter. *Human Development, 59*, 235–241. https://doi:10.1159 /000452289

Bjorklund, D. F. (2018). A metatheory for cognitive development (or "Piaget is dead" revisited). *Child Development, 89*, 2288–2302. https://doi.org/10.1111 /cdev.13019

Bjorklund, D. F. (2021). *How Children Invented Humanity: The Role of Development in Human Evolution*. New York, NY: Oxford University Press.

Bjorklund, D. F. (in press). Humans as a neotenous species. In M. Alemany-Oliver and R. W. Belk, (Eds.), *"Like a Child Would Do": A Multidisciplinary Approach to Childlikeness in Past and Current Societies*. Montreal: Universitas Press.

Bjorklund, D. F., & Bering, J. M. (2003). Big brains, slow development, and social complexity: The developmental and evolutionary origins of social cognition. In M. Brüne, H. Ribbert, and W. Schiefenhövel (Eds.), *The Social Brain: Evolutionary Aspects of Development and Pathology*. New York, NY: Wiley, pp. 133–151. https://doi.org/10.1002/0470867221.ch7

Bjorklund, D. F., & Causey, K. (2018). *Children's Thinking: Cognitive Development and Individual Differences* (6th ed.). Los Angeles, CA: Sage.

Bjorklund, D. F., Cormier, C., & Rosenberg, J. S. (2005). The evolution of theory of mind: Big brains, social complexity, and inhibition. In W. Schneider, R. Schumann-Hengsteler, and B. Sodian (Eds.), *Young Children's Cognitive Development: Interrelationships Among Executive Functioning, Working Memory, Verbal Ability and Theory of Mind*. Mahwah, NJ: Erlbaum, pp. 147–174.

Bjorklund, D. F., & Ellis, B. J. (2005). Evolutionary psychology and child development: An emerging synthesis. In B. J. Ellis and D. F. Bjorklund

(Eds.), *Origins of the Social Mind: Evolutionary Psychology and Child Development.* New York, NY: Guilford, pp. 3–18.

Bjorklund, D. F., & Ellis, B. J. (2014). Children, childhood, and development in evolutionary perspective. *Developmental Review, 34*, 225–264. https://doi .org/10.1016/j.dr.2014.05.005

Bjorklund, D. F., Ellis, B. J., & Rosenberg, J. S. (2007). Evolved probabilistic cognitive mechanisms: An evolutionary approach to gene × environment × development. In R. V. Kail (Ed.), *Advances in Child Development and Behavior*, Vol. 35. Oxford: Elsevier, pp. 1–39. https://doi.org/10.1016 /b978-0-12-009735-7.50006-2

Bjorklund, D. F., Gaultney, J. F., & Green, B. L. (1993). "I watch, therefore I can do": The development of meta-imitation over the preschool years and the advantage of optimism in one's imitative skills. In R. Pasnak and M. L. Howe (Eds.), *Emerging Themes in Cognitive Development*, Vol. 1. New York, NY: Springer-Verlag, pp. 79–102. https://doi.org/10.1007/978-1-4613-9223-1_4

Bjorklund, D. F., & Harnishfeger, K. K. (1995). The role of inhibition mechanisms in the evolution of human cognition and behavior. In F. N. Dempster and C. J. Brainerd (Eds.), *New Perspectives on Interference & Inhibition in Cognition.* New York, NY: Academic Press, pp 141–173. https://doi.org/10 .1016/B978-012208930-5/50006-4

Bjorklund, D. F., & Pellegrini, A. D. (2002). *The Origins of Human Nature: Evolutionary Developmental Psychology.* Washington, DC: American Psychological Association. https://doi.org/10.1037/10425-000

Bjorklund, D. F., Yunger, J. L., Bering, J. M., & Ragan, P. (2002). The generalization of deferred imitation in enculturated chimpanzees (*Pan troglodytes*). *Animal Cognition, 5*, 49–58. https://doi.org/10.1007/s10071-001-0124-5

Bloom, P., & Markson, L. (1998). Capacities underlying word learning. *Trends in Cognitive Science, 2*, 67–73. https://doi.org/10.1016/S1364-6613(98)01121-8

Bock, J., & Johnston, S. E. (2004). Play and subsistence ecology among the Okavango Delta Peoples of Botswana. *Human Nature, 15*, 63–81. https://doi .org/10.1007/s12110-004-1004-x

Bogin, B. (1999). *Patterns of Human Growth* (2nd ed.). Cambridge: Cambridge University Press.

Bogin, B. (2001). *The Growth of Humanity.* New York, NY: Wiley-Liss.

Bogin, B. (2003). The human pattern of growth and development in paleontological perspective. In J. L. Thompson, G. E. Krovitz, and A. J. Nelson (Eds.), *Patterns of Growth and Development in the Genus Homo.* Cambridge: Cambridge University Press, pp. 15–44. https://doi.org/10.1017 /cbo9780511542565

Bolk, L. (1926). On the problem of anthropogenesis. *Proc. Section Sciences Kon. Akad. Wetens. Amsterdam, 29*, 465–475.

Bornstein, M. H. (1989). Sensitive periods in development: Structural characteristics and causal interpretations. *Psychological Bulletin, 105*, 179–197. https://doi.org/10.1037/0033–2909.105.2.179

Bornstein, M. H. (2009). Toward a model of culture↔parent↔child transactions. In A. Sameroff (Ed.), *The Transactional Model of Development: How Children and Contexts Shape Each Other*. Washington, DC: American Psychological Association, pp. 139–161. https://doi.org/10.1037/11877–008

Bornstein, M. H., Haynes, O. M., O'Reilly, A. W., & Painter, K. M. (1996). Solitary and collaborative pretense play in early childhood: Sources of individual variation in the development of representational competence. *Child Development, 6*, 2910–2929. https://doi.org/10.2307/1131759

Bornstein, M. H., & Putnick, D. L. (2019). *The Architecture of the Child Mind: g, Fs, and the Hierarchical Model of Intelligence*. Abingdon: Routledge. https://doi.org/10.4324/9780429027307

Boulton, M. J., & Smith, P. K. (1990). Affective bias in children's perceptions of dominance relations. *Child Development, 61*, 221–229. https://doi.org/10.2307/1131061

Boyce, W. T. (2019). *The Orchid and the Dandelion: Why Some Children Struggle and How All Can Thrive*. New York, NY: Knopf.

Boyce, W. T., & Ellis, B. J. (2005). Biological sensitivity to context: I. An evolutionary-developmental theory of the origins and functions of stress reactivity. *Development and Psychopathology, 17*, 271–301. https://doi.org/10.1017/S0954579405050145

Brooks, R., & Meltzoff, A. N. (2002). The importance of eyes: How infants interpret adult looking behavior. *Developmental Psychology, 38*, 958–966. https://doi.org/10.1037/0012–1649.38.6.958

Bufill, E., Agustí, J., & Blesa, R. (2011). Human neoteny revisited: The case of synaptic plasticity. *American Journal of Human Biology, 23*, 729–739. https://doi.org/10.1002/ajhb.21225

Bushnell, I. W. R., Sai, F., & Mullin, J. T. (1989). Neonatal recognition of the mother's face. *British Journal of Developmental Psychology, 7*, 3–15. https://doi.org/10.1111/j.2044-835X.1989.tb00784.x

Buss, D. M., Haselton, M. G., Shackelford, T. K., Bleske, A. L., & Wakefield, J. C. (1998). Adaptations, exaptations, and spandrels. *American Psychologist, 53*, 533–548. https://doi.org/10.1037/0003-066X.53.5.533

Buttelmann, D., Carpenter, M., Call, J., & Tomasello, M. (2007). Enculturated chimpanzees imitate rationally. *Developmental Science, 10*, F31–F38. https://doi.org/10.1111/j.1467–7687.2007.00630.x

Buttelmann, D., Carpenter, M., Call, J., & Tomasello, M. (2008). Rational tool use and tool choice in human infants and great apes. *Child Development, 79*, 609–626. https://doi.org/10.1111/j.1467–8624.2008.01146.x

Buttelmann, D., Zmyj, N., Daum, M., & Carpenter, M. (2013). Selective imitation of in-group over out-group members in 14-month-olds. *Child Development, 84*, 422–428. https://doi.org/10.1111/j.1467–8624.2012.01860.x

Byrne, R. W. (2005). Social cognition: Imitation, imitation, imitation. *Current Biology, 15*, R489–R500. https://doi.org/10.1016/j.cub.2005.06.031

Byrnes, J. P., & Fox, N. A. (1998). The educational relevance of research in cognitive neuroscience. *Educational Psychology Review, 10*, 297–342. https://doi.org/10.1023/A:1022145812276

Caldera, Y. M., Huston, A. C., & O'Brien, M. (1989). Social interactions and play patterns of parents and toddlers with feminine, masculine, and neutral toys. *Child Development, 60*, 70–76. https://doi.org/10.2307/1131072

Call, J., & Tomasello, M. (1996). The effects of humans on the cognitive development of apes. In A. E. Russon, K. A. Bard, and S. T. Parker (Eds.), *Reaching into Thought: The Minds of the Great Apes.* New York, NY: Cambridge University Press, pp. 371–403.

Callaghan, T. C., Moll, H., Rakoczy, H., Warneken, F. L. U., Behne, T., & Tomasello, M. (2011). Early social cognition in three cultural contexts. *Monographs of the Society of Research in Child Development, 76*(2), 34–104. https://doi.org/10.1111/j.1540-5834.2011.00606.x

Cao-Lei, L., Massart, R., Suderman, M. J., Machnes, Z., Elgbeli, G., Laplante, D. P., Szyf, M., & King, S. (2014). DNA methylation signatures triggered by prenatal maternal stress exposure to a natural disaster: Project Ice Storm. *PLoS One, 9*(9), e107653. https://doi.org/10.1371/journal.pone.0107653

Carlson, S. M., White, R. E., & Davis-Unger, A. C. (2014). Evidence for a relationship between executive function and pretense representation in preschool children. *Cognitive Development, 29*, 1–16. https://doi.org/10.1016/j.cogdev.2013.09.001

Carpenter, M., Tomasello, M., & Striano, T. (1995). Joint attention and imitative learning in children, chimpanzees, and enculturated chimpanzees. *Social Development, 4*, 217–237. https://doi.org/10.1111/j.1467–9507.1995.tb00063.x

Carroll, S. B. (2005). *Endless Forms Most Beautiful: The New Science of Evo Devo.* New York, NY: Norton.

Casler, K., & Kelemen, D. (2005). Young children's rapid learning about artifacts. *Developmental Science, 8*, 472–480. https://doi.org/10.1111/j.1467–7687.2005.00438.x

Chance, M. R. A. (1962). Social behaviour and primate evolution. In M. F. A. Montagu (Ed.), *Culture and the Evolution of Man*. New York, NY: Oxford University Press, pp. 84–130.

Chang, L., Lu, H. J., Lansford, J. E., Skinner, A. T., Bornstein, M. H., Steinberg, L., Dodge, K. et al. (2019). Environmental harshness and unpredictability, life history, and social and academic behavior of adolescents in nine countries. *Developmental Psychology, 55*, 890–903. https://doi.org/10.1037/dev0000655

Chappell, J., Cutting, N., Apperly, I. A., & Beck, S. R. (2013). The development of tool manufacture in humans: What helps young children make innovative tools? *Philosophical Transactions of the Royal Society B: Biological Sciences, 368*, 20120409. https://doi.org/10.1098/rstb.2012.0409

Charlesworth, W. R. (1992). Darwin and developmental psychology: Past and present. *Developmental Psychology, 28*, 5–16. https://doi.org/10.1037/0012–1649.28.1.5

Charrier, C., Joshi, K., Coutinho-Budd, J., Kim, J-E., Lambert, N., de Marchena, J., Jin, W-L., Vanderhaeghen, P., Ghosh, A., Sassa, T., & Polleux, F. (2012). Inhibition of SRGAP2 function by its human-specific paralogs induces neoteny during spine maturation. *Cell, 149*, 923–935. https://doi.org/10.1016/j.cell.2012.03.034

Clay, Z. & Tennie, C. (2018). Is overimitation a uniquely human phenomenon? Insights from human children as compared to bonobos. *Child Development, 89*, 1535–1544. https://doi.org/10.1111/cdev.12857

Coen, E. (2000). *The Art of Genes: How Organisms Make Themselves*. Oxford: Oxford University Press.

Conradt, E. (2017). Using principles of behavioral epigenetics to advance research on early-life stress. *Child Development Perspective, 11*, 107–112. https://doi.org/10.1111/cdep.12219

Cook, M., & Mineka, S. (1989). Observational conditioning of fear to fear-relevant versus fear-irrelevant stimuli in rhesus monkeys. *Journal of Abnormal Psychology, 98*, 448–459. https://doi.org/10.1037/0021-843X.98.4.448

Corbit, J., Callaghan, T., & Svetlova, M. (2020). Toddlers' costly helping in three societies. *Journal of Experimental Child Psychology, 195*, 104841. https://doi.org/10.1016/j.jecp.2020.104841

Crabtree, J. W., & Riesen, A. H. (1979). Effects of the duration of dark rearing on visually guided behavior in the kitten. *Developmental Psychobiology, 12*, 291–303. https://doi.org/10.1002/dev.420120404

Cummins-Sebree, S. W., & Fragaszy, D. M. (2005). Choosing and using tools: Capuchins *(Cebus apella)* use a different metric than tamarins *(Saguinus oedipus). Journal of Comparative Psychology, 119*, 210–219. https://doi.org /10.1037/0735–7036.119.2.210

Cutting, N., Apperly, I. A., Chappell, C., & Beck, S. R. (2014). The puzzling difficulty of tool innovation: Why can't children piece their knowledge together? *Journal of Experimental Child Psychology, 125*, 110–117. https:// doi.org/10.1016/j.jecp.2013.11.010

de Beer, G. (1958). *Embryos and Ancestors* (3rd ed.). Oxford: Clarendon Press.

de Klerk, C. C. J. M., Bulgarelli, C., & Hamilton, A. (2019). Selective facial mimicry of native over foreign speakers in preverbal infants. *Journal of Experimental Child Psychology, 183*, 33–47. https://doi.org/10.1016/j .jecp.2019.01.015

Del Giudice, M., & Ellis, E. J. (2016). Evolutionary foundations of developmental psychopathology In D. Cicchetti (Ed.), *Developmental Psychopathology, Vol. 2: Developmental Neuroscience* (3rd ed.). New York, NY: Wiley, pp. 1–58. https://doi.org/10.1002/9781119125556.devpsy201

Del Giudice, M., Gangestad, S. W., & Kaplan, H. S. (2016). Life history theory and evolutionary psychology. In D. Buss (Ed.), *Evolutionary Psychology Handbook* (Vol. 2). New York, NY: Wiley, pp. 88–114.

DeLoache, J. S., & LoBue, V. (2009). The narrow fellow in the grass: Human infants associate snakes and fear. *Developmental Science, 12*, 201–207. https://doi.org/10.1111/j.1467–7687.2008.00753.x

Denenberg, V. H., & Rosenberg, K. M. (1967). Non-genetic transmission of information. *Nature, 216*, 549–550. https://doi.org/10.1038/216549a0

Dennett, D. (1987). *The Intentional Stance*. Cambridge, MA: The MIT Press.

Dennett, D. (1990). The interpretation of texts, people, and other artifacts. *Philosophy and Phenomenological Quarterly, 1* (Suppl.), 177–194. https:// doi.org/10.2307/2108038

Dennis, E. L., Jahanshad, N., McMahon, K. L., de Zubicaray, G. I., Martin, N. G., Hickie, I. B., Toga, A. W., Wright, M. J., and Thompson, P. M. (2013). Development of brain structural connectivity between ages 12 and 30: A 4-Tesladiffusion imaging study in 439 adolescents and adults. *NeuroImage, 64*, 671–684. https://doi.org/10.1016/j.neuroimage.2012.09.004

DeSilva, J. M. (2016). Brains, birth, bipedalism, and the mosaic evolution of the helpless infant. In W. R. Trevathan and K. R. Rosenberg (Eds.), *Costly and Cute: Helpless Infants and Human Evolution*. Santee Fe, MN: School for Advanced Research Press, pp. 67–86.

Dobzansky, T. (1973). Nothing in biology makes sense except in the light of evolution. *American Biology Teacher, 35*, 125–129. https://doi.org/10.2307 /4444260

Dunbar, R. I. M. (1995). Neocortex size and group size in primates: A test of the hypothesis. *Journal of Human Evolution, 28,* 287–296. https://doi.org/10.1006/jhev.1995.1021

Dunbar, R. I. M. (2003). The social brain: mind, language, and society in evolutionary perspective. *Annual Review of Anthropology, 32,* 163–181. https://doi.org/10.1146/annurev.anthro.32.061002.093158

Duncker, K. (1945). On problem-solving. *Psychological Monographs,* 58, i–113. https://doi.org/10.1037/h0093599

Dunham, Y., Baron, A. S., & Carey, S. (2011). Consequences of "minimal" group affiliations in children. *Child Development, 82,* 793–811. https://doi.org/10.1111/j.1467–8624.2011.01577.x

Elias, C. L., & Berk, L. E. (2002). Self-regulation in young children: Is there a role for executive function and pretense representation in preschool children. *Cognitive Development, 29,* 1–16. https://doi.org/10.1016/j.cogdev.2013.09.001

Ellis, B. J., Bianchi, J., Griskevicius, V., & Frankenhuis, W. E. (2017). Beyond risk and protective factors: An adaptation-based approach to resilience. *Perspectives on Psychological Science, 12,* 561–587. https://doi.org/10.1177/1745691617693054

Ellis, B. J., Boyce, W. T., Belsky, J., Bakermans-Kranenburg, M. J., & van IJzendoorn, M. H. (2011). Differential susceptibility to the environment: An evolutionary- neurodevelopmental theory. *Development and Psychopathology, 23,* 7–28. https://doi.org/10.1017/S0954579410000611

Ellis, B. J., Del Giudice, M., Dishion, T. J., Figueredo, A. J., Gray, P., Griskevicius, V., Hawley, P. H., Jacobs, W. J., James, J., Volk, A. A., & Wilson, D. S. (2012). The evolutionary basis of risky adolescent behavior: Implications for science, policy, and practice. *Developmental Psychology, 48,* 598–623. https://doi.org/10.1037/a0026220

Ellis, B. J., Figueredo, A. J., Brumbach, B. H., & Schlomer, G. L. (2009). Fundamental dimensions of environmental risk: The impact of harsh versus unpredictable environments on the evolution and development of life history strategies. *Human Nature, 20,* 204–268. https://doi.org/10.1007/s12110-009-9063-7

Ellis, B. J., Shirtcliff, E. A., Boyce, W. T., Deardorff, J., & Essex, M. J. (2011). Quality of early family relationships and the timing and tempo of puberty: Effects depend on biological sensitivity to context. *Development and Psychopathology, 23,* 85–99. https://doi.org/10.1017/S0954579410000660

Ellis, B. J., Volk, A. A., Gonzalez, J.-M., Embry, D. D. (2016). The meaningful roles intervention: An evolutionary approach to reducing bullying and increasing prosocial behavior. *Journal of Research on Adolescence, 26,* 622–637. https://doi.org/10.1111/jora.12243

Engelmann, J., Rapp, D., Herrmann, E., & Tomasello, M. (2018). Concern for group reputation increases prosociality in young children. *Psychological Science, 29*, 181–190. https://doi.org/10.1177/0956797617733830

Fabes, R. A., Fultz, J., Eisenberg, N., May-Plumlee, T., & Christopher, F. S. (1989). Effects of rewards on children's prosocial motivation: A socialization study. *Developmental Psychology, 25*, 509–515. https://doi.org/10.1037/0012-1649.25.4.509

Farroni, T., Csibra, G., Simion, F., & Johnson, M. H. (2002). Eye contact detection in humans from birth. *PNAS, 99*, 9602–9605. https://doi.org/10.1073/pnas.152159999

Francis, D. D., Diori, J., Liu, D., & Meaney, M. J. (1999). Nongenomic transmission across generations in maternal behavior and stress response in the rat. *Science, 286*, 1155–1158. https://doi.org/10.1126/science.286.5442.1155

Frankenhuis, W. E., de Vries, S. A., Bianchi, J. M., & Ellis, B. J. (2019). Hidden talents in harsh conditions? A preregistered study of memory and reasoning about social dominance. *Developmental Science*, e12835. https://doi.org/10.1111/desc.12835

Franklin, P., & Volk, A. A. (2018). A review of infants' and children's facial cues' influence on adults' perceptions and behaviors. *Evolutionary Behavioral Sciences, 12*, 296–321. https://doi.org/10.1037/ebs0000108

Garon, N., Bryson, S. E., & Smith, I. M. (2008). Executive function in preschoolers: A review using an integrative framework. *Psychological Bulletin, 134*, 31–60. https://doi.org/10.1037/0033-2909.134.1.31

Garstang, W. (1922). The theory of recapitulation: A critical restatement of the Biogenetic Law. *Proceedings of the Linnean Society of London: Zoology 35*, 81–101. https://doi.org/10.1111/j.1096-3642.1922.tb00464.x

Gava, L., Valenza, E., Turati, C., & de Schonen, S. (2008). Effect of partial occlusion on newborns' face preference and recognition. *Developmental Science, 11*, 563–574. https://doi.org/10.1111/j.1467-7687.2008.00702.x

Geary, D. C. (1995). Reflections of evolution and culture in children's cognition: Implications for mathematical development and instruction. *American Psychologist, 50*, 24–37. https://doi.org/10.1037/10871-000

Geary, D. C. (2005). *The Origin of Mind: Evolution of Brain, Cognition, and General Intelligence*. Washington, DC: American Psychological Association. https://doi.org/10.1037/10871–000

Geary, D. C. (2021). *Male, Female: The Evolution of Human Sex Differences (3rd ed.)*. Washington, DC: American Psychological Association.

Geary, D. C., & Berch, D. B. (Eds.). (2016). *Evolutionary Perspectives on Education and Child Development*. New York, NY: Springer. https://doi.org/10.1007/978–3-319–29986-0

Geary, D. C., & Bjorklund, D. F. (2000). Evolutionary developmental psychology. *Child Development, 71*, 57–65. https://doi.org/10.1111/1467–8624.00118

Gellén, K., & Buttelmann, D. (2019). Rational imitation declines within the second year of life: Changes in the function of imitation. *Journal of Experimental Child Psychology, 185*, 148–163. https://doi.org/10.1016/j.jecp.2019.04.019

German, T. P., & Johnson, S. C. (2002). Function and the origins of the design stance. *Journal of Cognition and Development, 3*, 279–300. https://doi.org/10.1207/S15327647JCD0303_2

Giedd, J. N. (2015). Risky teen behavior is drive by an imbalance in brain development. *Scientific American, 312*(6), 33–37. https://doi.org/10.1038/scientificamerican0615-32

Giedd, J. N., Bluenthal, J., Jeffries, N. O., Castellanos, F. X., Liu, H., Zijdenbos, A., Paus, T., Evans, A. C, & Rapoport, J. L. (1999). Brain development during childhood and adolescence: A longitudinal MRI study. *Nature Neuroscience, 2*, 861–863. https://doi.org/10.1038/13158

Gilad, Y., Oshlack, A., Smyth, G. K., Speed, T. P., & White, K. P. (2006). Expression profiling in primates reveals a rapid evolution of human transcription factors. *Nature, 440*, 242–245. https://doi.org/10.1038/nature04559

Gilissen, R., Bakermans-Kranenburg, M. J., van IJzendoorn, M. H., & Linting, M. (2008). Electrodermal reactivity during the Trier Social Stress Test for children: Interaction between the serotonin transporter polymorphism and children's attachment representation. *Developmental Psychobiology, 50*, 615–625. https://doi.org/10.1002/dev.20314

Glocker, M. L., Langleben, D. D., Ruparel, K., Loughead, J. W., Gur, R. C., & Sachser, N. (2009). Baby schema in infant faces induces cuteness perception and motivation for caretaking in adults. *Ethology, 115*, 257–263. https://doi.org/10.1111/j.1439-0310.2008.01603.x

Goldhaber, D. (2012). *The Nature-Nurture Debates: Bridging the Gaps*. Cambridge: Cambridge University Press. https://doi.org/10.1017/CBO9781139022583

Gómez, J-C., & Martín-Andrade, B. (2005). Fantasy play in apes. In A. D. Pellegrini and P. K. Smith (Eds.), *The Nature of Play: Great Apes and Humans*. New York, NY: Guilford Press, pp. 139–172.

Gopnik, A., & Meltzoff, A. N. (1997). *Words, Thoughts, and Theories*. Cambridge, MA: MIT Press.

Gottlieb, G. (1976). The roles of experience in the development of behavior and the nervous system. In G. Gottlieb (Ed.), *Neural and Behavioral Plasticity*. New York, NY: Academic Press, pp. 25–54. https://doi.org/10.1016/B978-0–12-609303–2.50008-X

Gottlieb, G. (1987). The developmental basis of evolutionary change. *Journal of Comparative Psychology, 101*, 262–271. https://doi.org/10.1037/0735-7036.101.3.262

Gottlieb, G. (1992). *Individual Development and Evolution: The Genesis of Novel Behavior.* New York, NY: Oxford University Press.

Gottlieb, G. (1997). *Synthesizing Nature-Nurture: Prenatal Roots of Instinctive Behavior.* Mahwah, NJ: Erlbaum.

Gottlieb, G. (2007). Probabilistic epigenesis. *Developmental Science, 10*, 1–11. https://doi.org/10.1111/j.1467–7687.2007.00556.x

Gottlieb, G., Wahlsten, D., & Lickliter, R. (2006). The significance of biology for human development: A developmental psychobiological systems view. In R. M. Lerner (Vol. Ed.), *Theoretical Models of Human Development*, Vol. 1, in W. Damon and R. M. Lerner (Gen. Eds.), *Handbook of Child Psychology* (6th ed.). New York, NY: Wiley, pp. 210–257. https://doi.org/10.1002/9780470147658.chpsy0105

Gould, S. J. (1977). *Ontogeny and Phylogeny.* Cambridge, MA: Harvard University Press.

Gray, P. (2016). Children's natural ways of educating themselves still works: Even for the three Rs. In D. C. Geary and D. B. Berch (Eds.), *Evolutionary Perspectives on Education and Child Development.* New York, NY: Springer, pp. 66–94. https://doi.org/10.1007/978–3-319–29986-0_3

Gredlein, J. M., & Bjorklund, D. F. (2005). Sex differences in young children's use of tools in a problem-solving task: The role of object-oriented play. *Human Nature, 16*, 211–232. https://doi.org/10.1007/s12110-005–1004-5

Greve, W., & Thomsen, T. (2016). Evolutionary advantages of free play during childhood. *Evolutionary Psychology*, 14, 1–9. https://doi.org/10.1177/1474704916675349

Greve, W., Thomsen, T., & Dehio, C. (2014). Does playing pay? The fitness-effect of free play during childhood. *Evolutionary Psychology, 12*, 434–447. https://doi.org/10.1177/147470491401200210

Griffey, J. A. F., & Little, A. C. (2014). Infants' visual preferences for facial traits associated with adult attractiveness judgments: Data from eye-tracking. *Infant Behavior and Development, 37,* 268–275. https://doi.org/10.1016/j.infbeh.2014.03.001

Groos, K. (1898/1975). *The Play of Animals.* New York, NY: Appleton. https://doi.org/10.1037/12894–000

Gruber, T., Deschenaux, A., Frick, A., & Clément, F. (2019). Group membership influences more social identification than social learning or overimitation in children. *Child Development, 90*, 728–745. https://doi.org/10.1111/cdev.12931

Haith, M. M. (1966). The response of the human newborn to visual movement. *Journal of Experimental Child Psychology, 3*, 235–243. https://doi.org/10.1016/0022–0965(66)90067–1

Hamann, K., Warneken, F., Greenberg, J. R., & Tomasello, M. (2011). Collaboration encourages equal sharing in children but not in chimpanzees. *Nature, 476*, 328–331. https://doi.org/10.1038/nature10278

Hamlin, J. K., Mahajan, N., Liberman, Z., & Wynn, K. (2013). Not like me = bad: Infants prefer those who harm dissimilar others. *Psychological science, 24*, 589–594. https://doi.org/10.1177/0956797612457785

Hare, B. (2017). Survival of the friendliest: *Homo sapiens* evolved via selection for prosociality. *Annual Review Psychology, 68*, 155–186. https://doi.org/10.1146/annurev-psych-010416–044201

Heimann, M. (1989). Neonatal imitation gaze aversion and mother-infant interaction. *Infant Behavior and Development, 12*, 495–505. https://doi.org/10.1016/0163–6383(89)90029–5

Henrich, J., Heine, S. J., & Norenzayan, A. (2010). The weirdest people in the world. *Behavioral and Brain Sciences, 33*, 61–135. https://doi.org/10.1017/S0140525X0999152X

Hepach, R. (2016). Prosocial arousal in children. *Child Development Perspectives, 11*, 50–55. https://doi.org/10.1111/cdep.12209

Hernández Blasi, C., & Bjorklund, D. F. (2003). Evolutionary developmental psychology: A new tool for better understanding human ontogeny. *Human Development, 46*, 259–281. https://doi.org/10.1159/000071935

Hernández Blasi, C., Bjorklund, D. F., Agut, S., Lozano, F., & Martínez, M. A. (July, 2018). *Vocal cues as signaling behavior in early childhood*. 30th Annual Meeting of the Human Behavior and Evolution Society, Amsterdam, The Netherlands.

Hernández-Blasi, C., Bjorklund, D. F., & Ruiz Soler, M. (2015). Cognitive cues are more compelling than facial cues in determining adults' reactions towards young children. *Evolutionary Psychology, 13*, 511–530. https://doi.org/10.1177/147470491501300212

Herrmann, E., Call, J., Hernandez-Lloreda, M., Hare, B., & Tomasello, M. (2007). Humans have evolved specialized skills of social cognition: The cultural intelligence hypothesis. *Science, 317*, 1360–1366. https://doi.org/10.1126/science.1146282

Hewlett, B. S., Berl, R. E. W., & Roulette, C. J. (2016). Teaching and over-imitation among Aka hunter-gatherers. In H. Terashima and B. Hewlett (Eds.), *Social Learning and Innovation in Contemporary Hunter-Gatherers*. Tokyo: Springer, pp. 35–45. https://doi.org/10.1007/978-4-431-55997-9_3

Hill, K., & Kaplan, H. (1999). Life history traits in humans: Theory and empirical studies. *Annual Review of Anthropology, 28*, 397–430. https://doi.org/10.1146/annurev.anthro.28.1.397

Hoehl, S., Keupp, S., Schleihauf, H., McGuigan, N., Buttelmann, D., & Whiten, A. (2019). 'Overimitation': A review and appraisal of a decade of research. *Developmental Review, 51*, 90–108. https://doi.org/10.1016/j.evolhumbehav.2016.12.001

Hood, B. (2014). *The Domesticated Brain*. London: Pelican.

Horner, V., & Whiten, A. (2005). Causal knowledge and imitation/emulation switching in chimpanzees (*Pan troglodytes*) and children (*Homo sapiens*). *Animal Cognition, 8*, 164–181. https://doi.org/10.1007/s10071-004-0239-6

House, B. R., Silk, J. B., Henrich, J., Barrett, H. C., Scelza, B. A., Boyette, A. H., Hewlett, B. S., & Laurence, S. (2013). Ontogeny of prosocial behavior across diverse societies. *PNAS, USA, 110*, 14586–14591. https://doi.org/10.1016/j.jecp.2017.12.014

House, B. R., & Tomasello, M. (2018). Modeling social norms increasingly influences costly sharing in middle childhood. *Journal of Experimental Child Psychology, 171*, 84–98. https://doi.org/10.1016/j.jecp.2017.12.014

Hubel, D. H., & Wiesel, T. N. (1962). Receptive fields, binocular interaction and functional architecture in the cat's visual cortex. *Journal of Physiology, 160*, 106–154. https://doi.org/10.1113/jphysiol.1962.sp006837

Ingram, G. (2014). From hitting to tattling to gossip: An evolutionary rationale for the development of indirect aggression. *Evolutionary Psychology, 12*, 343–363. https://doi.org/10.1177/147470491401200205

Ingram, G., & Bering, J. M. (2010). Children's tattling: A developmental precursor to gossip? *Child Development, 81*, 945–957. https://doi.org/10.1111/j.1467-8624.2010.01444.x

Joffe, T. H. (1997). Social pressures have selected for an extended juvenile period in primates. *Journal of Human Evolution, 32*, 593–605. https://doi.org/10.1006/jhev.1997.0140

Jordan, J. J., McAuliffe, K., & Warneken, F. (2014). Development of in-group favoritism in children's third-party punishment of selfishness. *PNAS, 111*, 12710–12715. https://doi.org/10.1073/pnas.1402280111

Keeley, L. H. (1996). *War Before Civilization: The Myth of the Peaceful Savage*. New York, NY: Oxford University Press.

Kelly, D. J., Liu, S., Lee, K., Quinn, P. C., Pascalis, O., Slater, A. M., & Ge, L. (2009). Development of the other-race effect in infancy: Evidence toward universality? *Journal of Experimental Child Psychology, 104*, 105–114. https://doi.org/10.1016/j.jecp.2009.01.006

Kenny, P., & Turkewitz, G. (1986). Effects of unusually early visual stimulation on the development of homing behavior in the rat pup. *Developmental Psychobiology, 19*, 57–66. https://doi.org/10.1002/dev.420190107

Kenward, B. (2012). Over-imitating preschoolers believe unnecessary actions are normative and enforce their performance by a third party. *Journal of Experimental Child Psychology, 112*, 195–207. https://doi.org/10.1016/j.jecp.2012.02.006

Kertes, D. A., Kamin, H. S., Hughes, D. A., Rodney, N. C., Bhatt, S., & Mulligan, C. J. (2016). Prenatal maternal stress predicts methylation of genes regulating the hypothalamic-pituitary-adrenocortical system in mothers and newborns in the Democratic Republic of Congo. *Child Development, 87*, 61–72. https://doi.org/10.1111/cdev.12487

Keupp, S., Behne, T., & Rakoczy, H. (2013). Why do children overimitate? Normativity is crucial. *Journal of Experimental Child Psychology, 116*, 392–406. https://doi.org/10.1016/j.jecp.2013.07.002

Kochanska, G. (1993). Toward a synthesis of parental socialization and child temperament in early development of conscience. *Child Development, 64*, 325–347. https://doi.org/10.2307/1131254

Konner, M. (2010). *The Evolution of Childhood: Relationships, Emotions, Mind*. Cambridge, MA: Belknap Press.

Koomen, R., Grueneisen, S., & Herrmann, E. (2020). Children delay gratification for cooperative ends. *Psychological Science, 31*, 139–148. https://doi.org/10.1177/0956797619894205

Kringelbach, M. L., Stark, E. A., Alexander, C., Bornstein, M. H., & Stein, A. (2016). On cuteness: Unlocking the parental brain and beyond. *Trends in Cognitive Science, 20*, 545–558. https://doi.org/10.1016/j.tics.2016.05.003

Lancy, D. (2015). *The Anthropology of Childhood* (2nd ed.). Cambridge: Cambridge University Press.

Lancy, D. (2020). *Child Helpers: A Multidisciplinary Perspective*. Cambridge Elements (K. D. Keith, Ed.). New York, NY: Cambridge University Press. https://doi.org/10.1017/9781108769204

Langlois, J., Ritter, J., Casey, R., & Sawin, D. (1995). Infant attractiveness predicts maternal behavior and attitudes. *Developmental Psychology, 31*, 464–472. https://doi.org/10.1037/0012-1649.31.3.464

Le Grand, R., Mondloch, C. J., Maurer, D., & Brent, H. P. (2001). Early visual experience and face processing. *Nature, 410*, 890. https://doi.org/10.1038/35073749

Legare, C. H., & Nielsen, M. (2015). Imitation and innovation: The dual engines of cultural learning. *Trends in Cognitive Sciences, 19*, 688–699. https://doi.org/10.1016/j.tics.2015.08.005

Lewin, K. (1943). Psychology and the process of group living. *Journal of Social Psychology, 17*, 113–131. https://doi.org/10.1080/00224545.1943.9712269

Lew-Levy, S., Kissler, S. M., Boyette, A. H., Crittenden, A. N., Mabulla, I. A., & Hewlett, B. S. (2020). Who teaches children to forage? Exploring the primacy of child-to-child teaching among Hadza and BaYaka hunter-gatherers of Tanzania and Congo. *Evolution and Human Behavior, 41*, 12–22. https://doi.org/10.1016/j.evolhumbehav.2019.07.003

Lewkowicz, D. (2011). The biological implausibility of the nature–nurture dichotomy and what it means for the study of infancy. *Infancy, 16*, 331–367. https://doi.org/10.1111/j.1532–7078.2011.00079.x

Lickliter, R. (1990). Premature visual stimulation accelerates intersensory functioning in bobwhite quail neonates. *Developmental Psychobiology, 23*, 15–27. https://doi.org/10.1002/dev.420230103

Lillard, A. S., Lerner, M. D., Hopkins, E. J., Dore, R. A., Smith, E. D., & Palmquist, C. M. (2013). The impact of pretend play on children's development: A review of the evidence. *Psychological Bulletin, 139*, 1–34. https://doi.org/10.1037/a0029321

Liszkowski, U., Carpenter, M., Striano, T., & Tomasello, M. (2006). 12- and 18-month-olds point to provide information for others. *Journal of Cognition and Development, 7*, 173–187. https://doi.org/10.1207/s15327647jcd0702_2

Liszkowski, U., Carpenter, M., & Tomasello, M. (2007). Pointing out new news, old news, and absent referents at 12 months of age. *Developmental Science, 10*, F1–F7. https://doi.org/10.1111/j.1467–7687.2006.00552.x

Liu, X., Somel, M., Tang, L., Yan, Z., Jiang, X., Guo, S., Yuan, Y., He, L., Oleksiak, A. Zhang, Y., Li, N., Hu, Y., Chen, W., Qiu, Z., Pääbo, S., & Khaitovich, P. (2012). Extension of cortical synaptic development distinguishes humans from chimpanzees and macaques. *Genome Research, 22*, 611–622. https://doi.org/10.1101/gr.127324.111

LoBue, V., & Adolph, K. E. (2019). Fear in infancy: Lessons from snakes, spiders, heights, and strangers. *Psychological Bulletin, 55*, 1889–1907. https://doi.org/10.1037/dev0000675

Lockhart, K. L., Chang, B., & Tyler, S. (2002). Young children's belief about the stability of traits: Protective optimism. *Child Development, 73*, 1408–1430. https://doi.org/10.1111/1467–8624.00480

Lockhart, K. L., Goddu, M. K., & Keil, F. C. (2017). Overoptimism about future knowledge: Early arrogance? *Journal of Positive Psychology, 12*, 36–46. https://doi.org/10.1080/17439760.2016.1167939

Lockman, J. J. (2000). A perception-action perspective on tool use development. *Child Development, 71*, 137–144. https://doi.org/10.1111/1467-8624.00127

Lorenz, K. (1952). *King Solomon's Rings*. New York, NY: Crowell. https://doi .org/10.1111/j.1439-0310.1943.tb00655.x

Lorenz, K. Z. (1943). Die angeboren Formen moglicher Erfahrung [The innate forms of possible experience]. *Zeitschrift fur Tierpsychologie, 5*, 233–409. https://doi.org/10.1111/j.1439–0310.1943.tb00655.x

Lucion, M. K., Oliveira, V., Bizarro, L., Bischoff, R., Pelufo Silveria, P., & Kauer-Sant'Anna, M. (2017). Attentional bias toward infant faces: Review of the adaptive and clinical relevance. *International Journal of Psychology, 114*, 1–8. https://doi.org/10.1016/j.ijpsycho.2017.01.008

Lukianoff, G., & Haidt, J. (2018). *The Coddling of the American Mind: How Good Intentions and Bad Ideas are Setting up a Generation for Failure*. New York, NY: Penguin Press.

Lumey, L. H. (1992). Decreased birthweights in infants after maternal in utero exposure to the Dutch famine of 1944–45. *Paediatric and Perinatal Epidemiology, 6*, 240–253. https://doi.org/10.1111/j.1365–3016.1992.tb00764.x

Luo, L. Z., Li, H., & Lee, K. (2011). Are children's faces really more appealing than those of adults? Testing the baby schema hypothesis beyond infancy. *Journal of Experimental Child Psychology, 110*, 115–124. https://doi.org/10 .1016/j.jecp.2011.04.002

Macchi Cassia, V., Turati, C., & Simion, F. (2004). Can a nonspecific bias toward top-heavy patterns explain newborns' face preference? *Psychological Science, 15*, 379–383. https://doi.org/10.1111/j.0956–7976.2004.00688.x

Machluf, K., & Bjorklund, D. F. (May, 2016). *Physical immaturity in infants triggers greater empathy in adults*. Paper presented at meeting of the Association of Psychological Science, Chicago, IL.

Manuck, S. B., Craig, A. E., Flory, J. D., Halder, I., & Ferrell, R. E. (2011). Reported early family environment covaries with menarcheal age as a function of polymorphic variation in estrogen receptor-a. *Development and Psychopathology, 23*, 69–83. https://doi.org/10.1017/S0954579410000659

Marshall, P. J. (2015). Neuroscience, embodiment, and development. In W. F. Overton and P. C. M. Molenaar (Vol. Eds.), *Handbook of Child Psychology and Developmental Science* (R. M. Lerner, Gen. Ed.), Vol. 1. New York, NY: Wiley. https://doi.org/10.1002/9781118963418.childpsy107

Martin, C. L., Ruble, D. N., & Szkrybalo, J. (2002). Cognitive theories of early gender development. *Psychological Bulletin, 128*, 903–933. https://doi.org /10.1037/0033–2909.128.6.903

Maurer, D., & Lewis, T. L. (2013). Sensitive periods in visual development. In P. D. Zelazo (Ed.), *Oxford Handbook of Developmental Psychology*, Vol. 1. Oxford: Oxford University Press, pp. 202–234. https://doi.org/10.1093 /oxfordhb/9780199958450.013.0008

Maurer, D., Mondloch, C. J., & Lewis, T. L. (2007). Effects of early visual deprivation on perceptual and cognitive development. *Progress in Brain Research, 164*, 87–104. https://doi.org/10.1016/S0079-6123(07)64005-9

Mayr, E. (1982). *The Growth of Biological Thought: Diversity, Evolution, and Inheritance*. Cambridge, MA: Belknap Press.

Mayr, E., & Provine, W. B. (1980). *The Evolutionary Synthesis: Perspectives on the Unification of Biology*. Cambridge, MA: Harvard University Press. https://doi.org/10.4159/harvard.9780674865389

McAuley, T., & White, D. A. (2011). A latent variables examination of processing speed, response inhibition, and working memory during typical development. *Journal of Experimental Child Psychology, 108*, 152–166. https://doi.org/10.1016/j.jecp.2010.08.009

McClean, C. Y., Reno, P. L., Pollen, A. A., Bassan, A. I., Capellini, T. D., Guenther, C.,... Kingsley, D. M. (2011). Human-specific loss of regulatory DNA and the evolution of human-specific traits. *Nature, 471*, 216–219. https://doi.org/10.1038/nature09774

McGuigan, N., Makinson, J., & Whiten, A. (2011). From over-imitation to super-copying: Adults imitate causally irrelevant aspects of tool use with higher fidelity than young children. *British Journal of Psychology, 102*, 1–18. https://doi.org/10.1348/000712610X493115

McKinney, M. L., & McNamara, K. (1991). *Heterochrony: The Evolution of Ontogeny*. New York, NY: Plenum. https://doi.org/10.1007/978-1-4757-0773-1

Meaney, M. J. (2001). Maternal care, gene expression, and the transmission of individual differences in stress reactivity across generations. *Annual Review of Neuroscience, 24*, 1161–1192. https://doi.org/10.1146/annurev.neuro.24.1.1161

Meaney, M. J. (2010). Epigenetics and the biological definition of gene environment interactions. *Child Development, 81*, 41–79. https://doi.org/10.1111/j.1467-8624.2009.01381.x

Meaney, M. J. (2013). Epigenetics and the environmental regulation of the genome and its function. In D. Narvaez, J. Panksepp, A. N. Schore, and T. R. Gleason (Eds.), *Evolution, Early Experience and Human Development: From Research to Practice and Policy*. Oxford: Oxford University Press, pp. 99–128. https://doi.org/10.1093/acprof:oso/9780199755059.003.0006

Melas, P. A., Wei, Y., Wong, C. C., Sjöholm, L. K., Åberg, E., Mill, J., ... & Lavebratt, C. (2013). Genetic and epigenetic associations of MAOA and NR3C1 with depression and childhood adversities. *International Journal of Neuropsychopharmacology, 16*, 1513–1528. https://doi.org/10.1017/S1461145713000102

Meltzoff, A. N., & Moore, M. K. (1977). Imitation of facial and manual gestures by human neonates. *Science*, *198*, 75–78. https://doi.org/10.1126/science .897687

Merz, E. C., Harlé, K. M., Noble, K. G., & McCall, R. B. (2016). Executive function in previously institutionalized children. *Child Development Perspectives*, *10*, 105–110. https://doi.org/10.1111/cdep.12170

Miller, D. J., Duka, T., Stimpson, C. D., Schapiro, S. J., Baze, W. B., McArthur, M. J., Fobbs, A. J., Sousa, A. M. M., Šestan, N., Wildman, D. E., Lipovich, L., Kuzawa, C. W., Hof, P. R., & Sherwood, C. C. (2012). Prolonged myelination in human neocortical evolution. *PNAS*, *109*, 16480–16485. https:// doi.org/10.1073/pnas.1117943109

Mills, K. L., Goddings, A. L., Clasen, L. S., Giedd, J. N., & Blakemore, S. J. (2014). The developmental mismatch in structural brain maturation during adolescence. *Developmental Neuroscience*, *36*, 147–160. https://doi.org/10 .1159/000362328

Mittal, C., Griskevicius, V., Simpson, J. A., Sung, S., & Young, E. S. (2015). Cognitive adaptations to stressful environments: When childhood adversity enhances adult executive function. *Journal of Personality and Social Psychology*, 109, 604–621. https://doi.org/10.1037/pspi0000028

Mondloch, C. J., Lewis, T. M., Budreau, D. R., Maurer, D., Dannemiller, J. L., Benjamin R., Stephens, B. R., & Kleiner-Gathercoal, K. A. (1999). Face perception during early infancy. *Psychological Science*, *10*, 419–422. https:// doi.org/10.1111/1467–9280.00179

Montagu, A. (1989). *Growing Young* (2nd ed.). Grandy, MA: Bergin and Garvey.

Moore, D. D. (2015). *The Developing Genome: An Introduction to Behavioral Epigenetics*. New York, NY: Oxford University Press.

Morgan, D. K., & Whitelaw, E. (2008). The case for transgenerational epigen-etic inheritance in humans, *Mammalian Genome*, *19*, 394–397. https://doi .org/10.1007/s00335-008–9124-y

Morss, J. R. (1990). *The Biologising of Childhood: Developmental Psychology and the Darwinian Myth*. Hillsdale, NJ: Erlbaum.

Nagell, K., Olguin, K., & Tomasello, M. (1993). Processes of social learning in the tool use of chimpanzees (*Pan troglodytes*) and human children (*Homo sapiens*). *Journal of Comparative Psychology*, *107*, 174–186. https://doi.org /10.1037/0735–7036.107.2.174

Nagy, E. (2006). From imitation to conversation: The first dialogues with human neonates, *Infant and Child Development*, *15*, 223–232. https://doi .org/10.1002/icd.460

Nelson, C. A. III, Zeanah, C. H., Fox, N. A., Marshall, P. J., Smuke, A. T., & Guthrie, D. (2007). Cognitive recovery in socially deprived young children:

The Bucharest Early Intervention Program. *Science, 318*, 1937–1940. https://doi.org/10.1126/science.1143921

Nielsen, M. (2012). Imitation, pretend play, and childhood: Essential elements in the evolution of human culture? *Journal of Comparative Psychology, 126*, 170–181. https://doi.org/10.1037/a0025168

Nielsen, M. (2018). The social glue of cumulative culture and ritual behavior. *Child Development Perspectives, 12*, 264–268. https://doi.org/10.1111/cdep.12297

Nielsen, M., Haun, D., Kärtner, J., & Legare, C. H. (2017). The persistent sampling bias in developmental psychology: A call to action. *Journal of Experimental Child Psychology, 162*, 31–38. https://doi.org/10.1016/j.jecp.2017.04.017

Nielsen, M., Mushin, I., Tomaselli, K., & Whiten, A. (2014). Where culture takes hold: "Overimitation" and its flexible deployment in Western, Aboriginal, and Bushmen children. *Child Development, 85*, 2169–2184. https://doi.org/10.1111/cdev.12265

Nielsen, M., Mushin, B., Tomaselli, K., & Whiten, A. (2016). Imitation, collaboration, and their interaction among Western and indigenous Australian preschool children. *Child Development, 87*, 755–806. https://doi.org/10.1111/cdev.12504

Noonan, J. P. (2003). Regulatory DNAs and the evolution of human development. *Current Opinion in Genetics and Development, 19*, 557–564. https://doi.org/10.1016/j.gde.2009.10.002

Nussey, D. H., Postma, E., Gienapp, P., & Visser, M. E. (2005). Selection on heritable phenotypic plasticity in a wild bird population. *Science, 310*, 304–306. https://doi.org/10.1126/science.1117004

Obradović, J., Bush, N. R., Stamperdahl, J., Adler, N. E., & Boyce, W. T. (2010). Biological sensitivity to context: The interactive effects of stress reactivity and family adversity on socioemotional behavior and school readiness. *Child Development, 81*, 270–289. https://doi.org/10.1111/j.1467-8624.2009.01394.x

Öhman, A., Flykt, A., & Esteves, F. (2001). Emotion drives attention: Detecting the snake in the grass. *Journal of Experimental Psychology: General, 130*, 466–478. https://doi.org/10.1037/0096-3445.130.3.466

Olson, K. R., & Spelke, E. S. (2008). Foundations of cooperation in young children. *Cognition, 108*, 222–231. https://doi.org/10.1016/j.cognition.2007.12.003

Oostenbroek, J., Suddendorf, T., Nielsen, M., Redshaw, J., Kennedy-Costantini, S., Davis, J., . . . & Slaughter, V. (2016). Comprehensive longitudinal study challenges the existence of neonatal imitation in humans. *Current Biology, 26*, 1334–1338. https://doi.org/10.1016/j.cub.2016.03.047

Overton, W. F. (2015). Processes, relations, and relational-developmental-systems. In W. F. Overton and P. C. M. Molenaar (Eds.), *Handbook of child psychology and developmental science. Vol. 1: Theory and method* (7th ed.). Hoboken, NJ: Wiley, p. 9–62. https://doi.org/10.1002/9781118963418.childpsy102

Painter, R. C. Osmond, C., Gluckman, P. Hanson, M., Philips, D. I. W., & Roseboom, T. J. (2008). Transgenerational effects on prenatal exposure to the Dutch famine on neonatal adiposity and health in later life. *BJOG, 115,* 1243–1249. https://doi.org/10.1111/j.1471–0528.2008.01822.x

Parades, S. H., Ridout, K. K., Seifer, R., Armstrong, D. A., Marisit, C., McWilliams, M. A., & Tyrka, A. R. (2016). Methylation of the glucocorticoid receptor gene promoter in preschoolers: Link with internalizing behavior problems. *Child Development, 87,* 86–97. http://dx.doi.org/10.1111/cdev.12484

Pascalis, O., de Haan, M., & Nelson, C. A. (2002). Is face processing species-specific during the first year of life? *Science, 296,* 1321–1323. https://doi.org/10.1126/science.1070223

Pascalis, O., Scott, L. S., Kelly, D. J., Shannon, R. W., Nicholson, E., Coleman, M., & Nelson, C. A. (2005). Plasticity of face processing in infancy. *PNAS, 102,* 5297–5300. https://doi.org/10.1073/pnas.0406627102

Patterson, M. M., & Bigler, R. S. (2006). Preschool children's attention to environmental messages about groups: Social categorization and the origins of intergroup bias. *Child Development, 77,* 847–860. https://doi.org/10.1111/j.1467–8624.2006.00906.x

Pellegrini, A. D. (2013a). Object use in childhood: Development and possible functions. *Behaviour, 150,* 813–843. https://doi.org/10.1163/1568539X-00003086

Pellegrini, A. D. (2013b). Play. In P. Zelazo (Ed.), *Oxford Handbook of Developmental Psychology.* New York, NY: Oxford University Press, pp. 276–299.

Pellegrini, A. D., & Galda, L. (1982). The effects of thematic-fantasy play training on the development of children's story comprehension. *American Educational Research Journal, 19,* 443–452. https://doi.org/10.3102/00028312019003443

Pellegrini, A. D., & Smith, P. K. (1998). Physical activity play: The nature and function of neglected aspect of play. *Child Development, 69,* 577–598. https://doi.org/10.1111/j.1467–8624.1998.tb06226.x

Periss, V., & Bjorklund, D. F. (2011). Trials and tribulations of childhood: An evolutionary perspective. In C. Salmon and T. Shackelford (Eds.), *Oxford Handbook of Evolutionary Family Psychology.* Oxford: Oxford University Press, pp. 149–168. https://doi.org/10.1093/oxfordhb/9780195396690.013.0010

Petanjek, Z., Judaš, M., Šimić, G., Roko Rašin, M., Uylings, H. B. M., Rakic, P., & Kostović, I. (2011). Extraordinary neoteny of synaptic spines in the human prefrontal cortex. *PNAS, 108,* 13281–13286. https://doi.org/10.1073/pnas .1105108108

Plötner, M., Over, H., Carpenter, M., & Tomasello, M. (2015). The effects of collaboration and minimal-group membership on children's prosocial behavior, liking, affiliation, and trust. *Journal of Experimental Child Psychology, 139,* 161–173. https://doi.org/10.1016/j.jecp.2015.05.008

Portmann, A. (1990). *A Zoologist Looks at Humankind.* Judith Schaefer (trans.). New York, NY: Columbia University Press. (Originally published in 1944).

Prabhakar, S., Noonan, J. P., Pääbo, S., & Rubin, E. M. (2006). Accelerated evolution of conserved noncoding sequences in humans. *Science, 314,* 786. https://doi.org/10.1126/science.1130738

Quinn, P. C., Yahr, J., Kuhn, A., Slater, A. M., & Pascalis, O. (2002). Representation of the gender of human faces by infants: A preference for female. *Perception, 31,* 1109–1121. https://doi.org/10.1068/p3331

Raff, R. A. (1996). *The Shape of Life: Genes, Development, and the Evolution of Animal Form.* Chicago, IL: University of Chicago Press. https://doi.org/10 .7208/chicago/9780226256573.001.0001

Rakoczy, H., & Haun, D. (2020). Comparative cognition between. Children and animals. In S. Hupp and J. Jewell (Eds.), *Encyclopedia of Child and Adolescent Development.* New York, NY: Wiley. https://doi.org/10.1002 /9781119171492.wecad109

Redshaw, J., Nielsen, M., Slaughter, V., Kennedy-Costantini, S., Oostenbroek, J., Crimston, J., & Suddendorf, T. (2019). Individual differences in neonatal 'imitation' fail to predict early social cognitive behavior. *Developmental Science, 23,* e12892. https://doi.org/10.1111/desc .12892

Ressler, R. H. (1966). Inherited environmental influences on the operant behavior of mice. *Journal of Comparative and Physiological Psychology, 61,* 264–267. https://doi.org/10.1037/h0023140

Rheingold, H. (1982). Little children's participation in the work of adults: A nascent prosocial behavior. *Child Development, 53,* 114–125. https://doi .org/10.2307/1129643

Riedl, K., Jensen, K., Call, J. M., & Tomasello, M. (2012). No third-party punishment in chimpanzees. *PNAS, 109,* 14824–14829. https://doi.org/10 .1073/pnas.1203179109

Riedl, K., Jensen, K., Call, J. M., & Tomasello, M. (2015). Restorative justice in children. *Current Biology, 25,* 1731–1735. https://doi.org/10.1016/j .cub.2015.05.014

Robbins, E., & Rochat, P. (2011). Emerging signs of strong reciprocity in human ontogeny. *Frontiers in Psychology*, *353*, 1–14. https://doi.org/10.3389/fpsyg.2011.00353

Rochat, P. M., Dias, D. G., Guo, L., Broesch, T., Passos-Ferreira, C. Winning, A., & Berg, B. (2009). Fairness in distributive justice by 3- and 5-year-olds across seven cultures. *Journal of Cross-Cultural Psychology*, *40*, 416–442. https://doi.org/10.1177/0022022109332844

Romens, S. E., McDonald, J., Svaren, J., & Pollak, S. D. (2015). Associations between early Life stress and gene methylation in children. *Child Development*, *86*, 303–309. https://doi.org/10.1111/cdev.12270

Ruff, H. A., & Birch, H. G. (1974). Infant visual fixation: The effect of concentricity, curvilinearity, and number of directions. *Journal of Experimental Child Psychology*, *17*, 460–473. https://doi.org/10.1016/0022–0965(74)90056–3

Ruiz, A. M., & Santos, L. R. (2013). Understanding differences in the way human and non-human primates represent tools: The role of teleological-intentional information. In C. M. Sanz, J. Call, and C. Boesch (Eds.), *Tool Use in Animals: Cognition and Ecology*. Cambridge: Cambridge University Press, pp. 119–133. https://doi.org/10.1017/CBO9780511894800.008

Rutter, M., Beckett,C. Castle, J., Colvert, E., Kreppner, J., Mehta, M. et al. (2007). Effects of profound early institutional deprivation: An overview of findings from a UK longitudinal study of Romanian adoptee. *European Journal of Developmental Psychology*, *4*, 332–350. https://doi.org/10.1080/17405620701401846

Salapatek, P., & Kessen, W. (1966). Visual scanning of triangles by the human newborn. *Journal of Experimental Child Psychology*, *3*, 155–167. https://doi.org/10.1016/0022–0965(66)90090–7

Samek, A., Cowell, J. M., Cappelen, A. W., Cheng, Y., Contreras-Ibáñez, C., Gomez-Sicard, N., Gonzalez-Gadea, M. L., Huepe, D., Ibáñez, A., Lee, K., Malcolm-Smith, S., Salas, N., Selcuk, B., Tungodden, B., Wong, A., Zhou, X., & Decety. J. (2020). The development of social comparisons and sharing behavior across 12 countries. *Journal of Experimental Child Psychology*, *192*, 104778. https://doi.org/10.1016/j.jecp.2019.104778

Sanefuji, W., Wada, K., Yamamoto, T., Mohri, I., & Taniike, M. (2014). Development of preference for conspecific faces in human infants. *Developmental Psychology*, *50*, 979–985. https://doi.org/10.1037/a0035205

Schmidt, M. F., Rakoczy, H., Mietzsch, T., & Tomasello, M. (2016). Young children understand and defend the role of agreement in establishing arbitrary norms – but unanimity is key. *Child Development*, *87*, 612–626. https://doi.org/10.1111/cdev.12510

Schneider, W. (1985). Developmental trends in the metamemory-memory behavior relationship: An integrative review. In D. L. Forrest-Pressley, G. E. MacKinnon, and T. G. Waller (Eds.), *Cognition, Metacognition, and Human Performance, Vol. 1.* New York, NY: Academic Press, pp. 57–109.

Schneider, W. (1998). Performance prediction in young children: Effects of skill, metacognition and wishful thinking. *Developmental Science, 1,* 291–297. https://doi.org/10.1111/1467–7687.00044

Seligman, M. E. P. (1991). *Learned Optimism: How to Change Your Mind and your Life* (1st ed.). New York, NY: Free Press.

Senese, V. P., De Falco, S., Bornstein, M. H., Caria, A., Buffolino, S., & Venutti. P. (2013). Human infant faces provoke implicit positive affective responses in parents and non-parents alike. *PLoS One, 8,* e80379. https://doi .org/10.1371/journal.pone.0080379

Shepperd, J. A., Klein, W. M. P., Waters, E. A., & Weinstein, N. D. (2013). Taking stock of unrealistic optimism. *Perspectives on Psychological Science, 8,* 395–411. https://doi.org/10.1177/1745691613485247

Shin, H.-E., Bjorklund, D. F., & Beck, E. F. (2007). The adaptive nature of children's overestimation in a strategic memory task. *Cognitive Development, 22,* 197–212. https://doi.org/10.1016/j.cogdev.2006.10.001

Shutts, K., Kinzler, K. D., McKee, C., & Spelke, E. (2009). Social information guides infants' selection of foods. *Journal of Cognition and Development, 10,* 1–17. https://doi.org/10.1080/15248370902966636

Simpson, E. A., Miller, G. M., Ferrari, P. F., Suomi, S. J., & Paukner, A. (2016). Neonatal imitation and early social experience predict gaze following abilities in infant monkeys. *Scientific Reports, 6,* 20233. https://doi.org/10.1038 /srep20233

Simpson, J. A., Griskevicius, V., Kuo, S., Sung, S., & Collins, W. A. (2012). Evolution, stress, and sensitive periods: The influence of unpredictability in early versus late childhood on sex and risky behavior. *Developmental Psychology, 48,* 674–686. https://doi.org/10.1037/a0027293

Skulachev, V. P., Holtze, S., Vyssokikh, M. Y., Bakeeva, L. E., Skulachev, M. V., Markov, A. V., Hildebrandt, T. B., & Sadovnichii, V. A. (2017). Neoteny, prolongation of youth: From naked mole rats to "naked ape" (humans). *Physiological Review, 97,* 699–720. https://doi.org/10.1152/physrev .00040.2015

Slagt, M., Dubas, J. S., Deković, M., & van Aken, M. A. G. (2016). Differences in sensitivity to parenting depending on child temperament: A meta-analysis. *Psychological Bulletin, 142,* 1068–1110. https://doi.org/10.1037 /bul0000061

Smilansky, S. (1968). *The Effects of Sociodramatic Play on Disadvantaged Preschool Children*. New York, NY: Wiley.

Smith, P. K. (1982). Does play matter? Functional and evolutionary aspects of animal and human play. *Behavioral and Brain Sciences*, *5*, 139–184. https://doi.org/10.1017/S0140525X0001092X

Somel, M., Rohlfs, R., & Liu, X. (2014). Transcriptomic insights into human brain evolution: acceleration, neutrality, heterochrony. *Genetics & Development*, *29*, 110–119. https://doi.org/10.1016/j.gde.2014.09.001

Spear, L. P. (2000). Neurobehavioral changes in adolescence. *Current Directions in Psychological Science*, *9*, 111–114. https://doi.org/10.1111/1467-8721.00072

Spear, L. P. (2007). Brain development and adolescent behavior. In D. Coch, K. W. Fischer, and G. Dawson (Eds.), *Human Behavior, Learning, and the Developing Brain: Typical Development*. New York, NY: Guilford, pp. 362–396.

Spelke, E. S., & Kinzler, K. D. (2007). Core knowledge. *Developmental Science*, *10*, 89–96. https://doi.org/10.1111/j.1467-7687.2007.00569.x

Stearns, S. (1992). *The Evolution of Life Histories*. Oxford: Oxford University Press.

Stengelin, R., Hepach, R., & Haun, D. (2020a). Being observed increases overimitation in three diverse cultures. *Developmental Psychology*, *55*, 2630–2636. https://doi.org/10.1037/dev0000832

Stengelin, R., Hepach, R., & Haun, D. (2020b). Cross-cultural variation in how much, but not whether, children overimitate. *Journal of Experimental Child Psychology*, *193*, 104796. https://doi.org/10.1016/j.jecp.2019.104796

Stenhouse, D. (1974). *The Evolution of Intelligence: A General Theory and Some of its Implications*. London: Allen and Unwin.

Stipek, D. (1981). Children's perceptions of their own and their classmates' ability. *Journal of Experimental Child Psychology*, *73*, 404–410. https://doi.org/10.1037/0022-0663.73.3.404

Stipek, D. (1984). Young children's performance expectations: Logical analysis or wishful thinking? In J. G. Nicholls (Ed.), *Advances in Motivation and Achievement: Vol. 3. The Development of Achievement Motivation*. Greenwich, CT: JAI, pp. 107–136.

Stright, A. D., Gallagher, K. C., & Kelley, K. (2008). Infant temperament moderates relations between maternal parenting in early childhood and children's adjustment in first grade. *Child Development*, *79*, 186–200. https://doi.org/10.1111/j.1467-8624.2007.01119.x

Sumner, J. A., McLaughlin, K. A., Walsh, K., Sheridan, M. A., & Koenen, K. C. (2015). Caregiving and 5-HTTLPR genotype predict adolescent physiological stress reactivity: Confirmatory tests of gene x environment interactions. *Child Development, 86*, 985–994. https://doi.org/10.1111/cdev.12357

Szepsenwol, O., Griskevicius, V., Simpson, J. A., Young, E. S., Fleck, C., & Jones, R. E. (2018). The effect of predictable early childhood environments on sociosexuality in early adulthood. *Evolutionary Behavioral Sciences, 11*, 131–145. https://doi.org/10.1037/ebs0000082

Tajfel, H., Billig, M. G., Bundy, R. P., & Flament, C. (1971). Social categorization and intergroup behaviour. *European Journal of Social Psychology, 1*, 149–178. https://doi.org/10.1002/ejsp.2420010202

Tasimi, A., & Wynn, K. (2016). Costly rejection of wrongdoers by infants and children. *Cognition, 151*, 76–79. https://doi.org/10.1016/j.cognition.2016.03.004

Tobi, E. W., Slieker, R. C., Stein, A. D., Suchiman, H. E. D., Slagboo, P. E., van Zwet, E. W., Heijmans, B. T., & Lumey, L. H. (2015). Early gestation as the critical time-window for changes in the prenatal environment to affect the adult human blood methylome. *International Journal of Epidemiology, 44*, 1211–1223. https://doi.org/10.1093/ije/dyv043

Tomasello, M. (2019). *Becoming Human: A Theory of Ontogeny.* Cambridge, MA: Belknap Press. https://doi.org/10.4159/9780674988651

Tomasello, M., & Carpenter, M. (2005). The emergence of social cognition in three young chimpanzees. *Monographs of the Society for Research in Child Development, 70*(1), vii–132. https://doi.org/10.1111/j.1540-5834.2005.00324.x

Tomasello, M., Savage-Rumbaugh, S., & Kruger, A. C. (1993). Imitative learning of actions on objects by children, chimpanzees, and enculturated chimpanzees. *Child Development, 64*, 1688–1705. https://doi.org/10.2307/1131463

Tomonaga, M., Tankak, M., Matsuzawa, T., Myowa-Yamakoshi, M., Kosugi, D., Mizuno, Y., Okamoto, S., Yamaguchi, M. K., & Bard, K. (2004). Development of social cognition in infant chimpanzees (*Pan troglodytes*): Face recognition, smiling, gaze, and the lack of triadic interactions. *Japanese Psychological Research, 46*, 227–235. https://doi.org/10.1111/j.1468-5584.2004.00254.x

Tottenham, N., Hare, T. A., Quinn, B. T., McCarry, T. W., Nurse, M., Gilhooly, T., Galvan, A., Davidson, M. C,... & Casey, B. J. (2010). Prolonged institutional rearing is associated with atypically large amygdala volume and difficulties in emotional regulation. *Developmental Science, 13*, 46–61. https://doi.org/10.1111/j.1467-7687.2009.00852.x

Tremblay, R. E., & Szyf, M. (2010). Developmental origins of chronic physical aggression and epigenetics. *Epigenomics, 2*, 495–499. https://doi.org/10.2217/epi.10.40

Trevathan, W. R., & Rosenberg, K. R. (2016). Human evolution and the helpless infant. In W. R. Trevathan and K. R. Rosenberg (Eds.), *Costly and Cute: Helpless Infants and Human Evolution.* Santee Fe, MN: School for advanced Research Press, pp. 1–28.

Trivers, R. (1972). Parental investment and sexual selection. In B. Campbell (Ed.), *Sexual Selection and the Descent of Man.* New York, NY: Aldine de Gruyter, pp. 136–179. https://doi.org/10.4324/9781315129266-7

Trut, L. (1999). Early canid domestication: The Farm-Fox Experiment. *American Scientist, 87,* 160. https://doi.org/10.1511/1999.2.160

Trut, L., Oskina, I., & Kharlamova, A. (2009). Animal evolution during domestication: The domesticated fox as a model. *BioEssays, 31,* 349–360. https://doi.org/10.1002/bies.200800070

Ulber, J., Hamann, K., & Tomasello, M. (2015). How 18- and 24-month-old peers divide resources among themselves. *Journal of Experimental Child Psychology, 140,* 228–244. https://doi.org/10.1016/j.jecp.2015.07.009

Ulber, J., Hamann, K., & Tomasello, M. (2016). Extrinsic rewards diminish costly sharing in 3-year-olds. *Child Development, 87,* 1192–1203. https://doi.org/10.1111/cdev.12534

Vaish, A., Hepach, R., & Tomasello, M. (2018). The specificity of reciprocity: Young children reciprocate more generously to those who *intentionally* benefit *them. Journal of Experimental Child Psychology, 167,* 336–353. https://doi.org/10.1016/j.jecp.2017.11.005

van IJzendoorn, M. H., Bakermans-Kranenburg, M. J., & Ebstein, R. P. (2011). Methylation matters in child development: Toward developmental behavioral epigenetics. *Child Development Perspectives, 5,* 305–310. https://doi.org/10.1111/j.1750-8606.2011.00202.x

Volk, A. A., & Atkinson, J. A. (2013). Infant and child death in the human environment of evolutionary adaptation. *Evolution and Human Behavior, 34,* 182–192. https://doi.org/10.1016/j.evolhumbehav.2012.11.007

Waddington, C. H. (1975). *The Evolution of an Evolutionist.* Ithaca, NY: Cornell University Press.

Waller, K. L., Volk, A., & Quinsey, V. L. (2004). The effect of infant fetal alcohol syndrome facial features on adoption preferences. *Human Nature, 15,* 101–117. https://doi.org/10.1007/s12110-004-1006-8

Warneken, F. (2015). Precocious prosociality: Why do young children help? *Child Development Perspectives, 9,* 1–6. https://doi.org/10.1111/cdep.12101

Warneken, F., Chen, F., & Tomasello, M. (2006). Cooperative activities in young children and chimpanzees. *Child Development, 77,* 640–663. https://doi.org/10.1111/j.1467-8624.2006.00895.x

Warneken, F., & Tomasello, M. (2006). Altruistic helping in human infants and young chimpanzees. *Science, 311*, 1301–1303. https://doi.org/10.1126/sci ence.1121448

Warneken, F., & Tomasello, M. (2008). Extrinsic rewards undermine altruistic tendencies in 20-month-olds. *Developmental Psychology, 44*, 1785–1788. https://doi.org/10.1037/a0013860

Warneken, F., & Tomasello, M. (2013). Parental presence and encouragement do not influence helping in young children. *Infancy, 18*, 345–368. https://doi .org/10.1111/j.1532–7078.2012.00120.x

Washburn, S. (1960). Tools and human evolution. *Scientific American, 203*, 3–15. https://doi.org/10.1038/scientificamerican0960-62

West-Eberhard, M. J. (2003). *Developmental Plasticity and Evolution.* New York, NY: Oxford University Press.

Whiten, A. (2019). Conformity and over-imitation: An integrative review of variant forms of hyper-reliance on social learning. *Advances in the Study of Behavior, 51*, 31–75.

Whiten A., & Erdal, D. (2014). The human socio-cognitive niche and its evolutionary origins. *Philosophical Transactions of the Royal Society B, 367*, 2119–2129. https://doi.org/10.1098/rstb.2012.0114

Wilson, D. S., Kauffman, R. A., & Purdy, M. S. (2011). A program for at-risk high school students informed by evolutionary science. *PLoS One, 6*(11), e27826. https://doi.org/10.1371/journal.pone.0027826

Witelson, S. F. (1987). Neurobiological aspects of language in children. *Child Development, 58*, 653–688. https://doi.org/10.2307/1130205

Witherington, D. C., & Lickliter, R. (2016). Integrating development and evolution in psychological science: Evolutionary developmental psychology, developmental systems, and explanatory pluralism. *Human Development, 59*, 200–234. https://doi.org/10.1159/000450715

Wobber, V., Herrmann, E., Hare, B., Wrangham, R., & Tomasello, M. (2014). Differences in the early cognitive development of children and great apes. *Developmental Psychobiology, 56*, 547–573. https://doi.org/10.1002/dev .21125

Wrangham, R. (2019). *Goodness Paradox: The Strange Relationship Between Virtue and Violence in Human Evolution.* New York, NY: Pantheon Books.

Wray, G. A. (2007). The evolutionary significance of *cis*-regulatory mutations. *Nature Review Genetics, 8*, 206–216. https://doi.org/10.1038/nrg2063

Yang, F., Choi, Y-J., Misch, A., Yang, X., & Dunham, Y. (2018). In defense of the commons: Young children negatively evaluate and sanction free riders. *Psychological Science, 29*, 1598–1611. https://doi.org/10.1177 /0956797618779061

Yeager, D. S., Dahl, R. E., & Dweck, C. S. (2018). Why interventions to influence adolescent behavior often fail but could succeed. *Perspectives on Psychological Science, 13*, 101–122. https://doi.org/10.1177/1745691617722620

Yeats, K. O., & Taylor, G. H. (2005). Neurobehavioral outcomes of mild head injury in children and adolescents. *Pediatric Rehabilitation, 8*, 5–16. https://doi.org/10.1080/13638490400011199

Zell, E., Strickhouser, J. E., Sedikides, C., & Alicke, M. D. (2020). The better-than-average effect in comparative self-evaluation: A comprehensive review and meta-analysis. *Psychological Bulletin, 146*, 118–149. https://doi.org/10.1037/bul0000218

Acknowledgment

I would like to thank Carlos Hernández Blasi and two anonymous reviewers for constructive comments on earlier drafts of this manuscript.

Cambridge Elements ☰

Child Development

Marc H. Bornstein
National Institute of Child Health and Human Development, Bethesda
Institute for Fiscal Studies, London
UNICEF, New York City
Marc H. Bornstein is an Affiliate of the *Eunice Kennedy Shriver* National Institute of Child Health and Human Development, an International Research Fellow at the Institute for Fiscal Studies (London), and UNICEF Senior Advisor for Research for ECD Parenting Programmes. Bornstein is President Emeritus of the Society for Research in Child Development, Editor Emeritus of *Child Development*, and founding Editor of *Parenting: Science and Practice.*

About the Series
Child development is a lively and engaging, yet serious and purposeful subject of academic study that encompasses myriad of theories, methods, substantive areas, and applied concerns. Cambridge Elements in Child Development proposes to address all these key areas, with unique, comprehensive, and state-of-the-art treatments, introducing readers to the primary currents of research and to original perspectives on, or contributions to, principal issues and domains in the field.

Cambridge Elements $\equiv$

Child Development

Elements in the Series

Printed in the United States
By Bookmasters